Happy days

Frances Neer

DANCING IN THE DARK

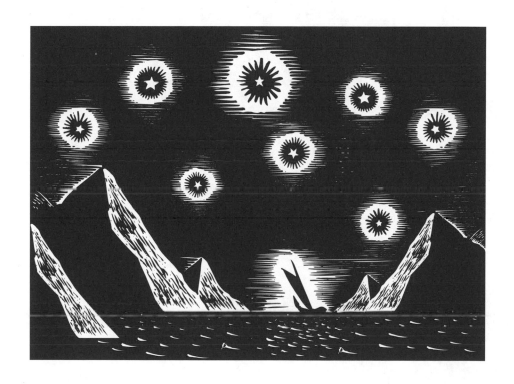

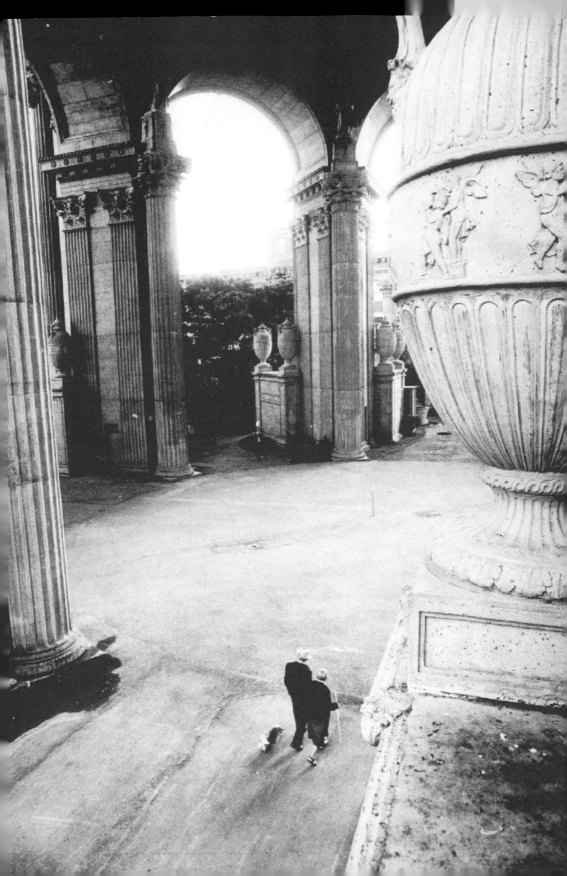

DANCING
IN
THE
DARK

FRANCES LIEF NEER

Wildstar Publishing
an imprint of
Rebecca House™

San Francisco

The proceeds from the sale of this book are donated to the William L. Neer Memorial Scholarship Fund, San Francisco State University Foundation, Programs in Visual Impairment. Recipients are pursuing credentials to teach individuals who are visually impaired.

Library of Congress Cataloging-in-Publication Data

Neer, Frances L., 1915-
      Dancing in the dark : when your sight begins to change / Frances
   L. Neer.
            p.   cm.
      ISBN 0-9637839-0-4:
      1. Visually handicapped—United States—Life skills guides.
      2. Blind—United States—Life skills guides.   I. Title.
      HV1795.N44   1994   93-23291
                                                                CIP

Wildstar Publishing, an imprint of Rebecca House™
1550 California Street, Suite 330
San Francisco, California 94109
[415] 752-1453

Design and production of text and cover:
Teutschel Design Services
Palo Alto, California

Photograph courtesy of San Francisco Examiner, Kim Komenich

Body copy is 13pt Bodoni set on 16pts of lead. Heads are Bodoni Bold Condensed. Paper: Glatfelter Thor Offset, Acid Free

Printed in the United States of America.
ISBN 0-9637839-0-4   SAN 247-1361
First Edition   10 9 8 7 6 5 4 3 2 1
Printed on recycled paper

DEDICATION

This book is lovingly dedicated to my ABC's:
my daughter Amy,
my son-in-law Bruce,
the memory of my beloved son Bill,
and to his daughter Christine.

Acknowledgements

Special thanks to these friends for their trust and encouragement:

Ronald Bansemer
Josephine Gregory
Joseph Alden Thompson
George S. Ladd Chapter - Telephone Pioneers of America

I thank the following friends for their expertise and professional opinions:

Catherine A. Fox
Dr. William Good
Susan Kroll
Christopher Lief
Ellen Lewis Lief
Louis Marracci
Dr. James Tulsky

The Photography Dept. of the San Francisco Examiner
Kim Komenich

and for the splendid editing by
Information Processing Services, Mt. Kisco, NY.

This book would never have come to fruition without
David Kenneth Waldman, Publisher
Wildstar Publishing, San Francisco.

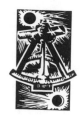

TABLE OF CONTENTS

FOREWORD

I was no more than four years old when I first noticed my grandmother's loss of vision. Somehow I understood that she needed her glasses in order to maneuver herself through her day. To me, she wasn't even awake until she had her glasses on. I remember shaking her and saying, "Granny, put your glasses on." For only then would she be able to make me breakfast or read me a story.

After the age of seven or eight I would take hold of her hand or arm, guiding her through a store to find particular items: kleenex, chocolate, milk . . . Somehow, without being told, I sensed she needed special help. And yet despite my understanding of her special needs, as a child I always recognized my grandmother as a capable, strong, and independent person.

As I have grown older and lived with her longer, I consider my grandmother's lack of sight in my own life and work. She tells me her greatest loss was not being able to see her family, and not being able to appreciate art. When I work on sculpture I think of how to make a piece worth feeling as well as seeing, and ask myself: How can this piece make sense to a person with a visual impairment?

I always remember this, especially when I work with clay. I want my grandmother to get something from my work, so I'll make "readable" faces or exaggerated textures. Touching the work is as important as seeing it. I also put on a blindfold in order to understand how people use their fingers as eyes.

My grandmother has given me the wonderful gift of recognizing peoples abilities instead of their disabilities.

Christine Neer
San Francisco, California
October, 1993

Chapter 1
WHEN YOUR SIGHT BEGINS TO CHANGE

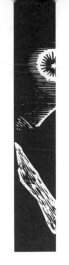

In 1980, when I knew that my sight was changing rather rapidly, I could still read. I could still get around without a white cane. I could still get on and off buses. I simply had to be careful. Little by little, as my sight continually diminished over the years, I found that I needed help.

My first sign of serious vision loss occurred one day when I was crossing a quiet street. I took off my glasses to wipe them and I said, "My goodness, I'm so lazy about keeping these glasses clean. They're such a blur." I wiped and put them back on, but the blur was still there. I didn't realize that this was a significant sign of a serious deterioration. At that point I should have run, not walked, to the nearest ophthalmologist, but I didn't. I knew no better. However, I eventually did get to an ophthalmologist because something else happened within a month or two of the dirty glasses incident.

I like to play tennis, but I was such a poor tennis player that I would never play a friendly game with anybody, and so I hired a "gigolo," a young man I would get out on the tennis court once a week to "play" tennis. Now, I'd be whacking at the ball the best I could and he'd be very patient with me, he was being paid for it. But one day I discovered that I was missing all the balls that were hit over to my right. And that's what finally woke me up and made me realize that there must be something wrong with my eyesight. That's finally what took me to the doctor.

Most of the time, Mother Nature is kind to us and changing sight is a very slow process. But sometimes change comes down on us swiftly and irrevocably. The following is what happened to me, with an anecdote to go with it. I traveled up to the Shakespeare festival in Ashland, Oregon and spent a few days there with a group of people to go to the theater. Well, two things happened. I discovered I couldn't see the stage anymore. Even worse, I found that I wasn't able to distinguish the faces of my acquaintances in the group. So I found myself retreating from them. They didn't know me well enough to understand what was happening, they simply thought I was a quiet or a shy person. But I wasn't. I was suffering great distress because I thought that I could no longer be the social animal that I had once been. When I came home I took myself to my bed and sobbed and despaired for three whole days, feeling that my life had come to an end. But on the fourth morning I arose and said, "Enough. I'm going downtown to get a cappuccino maker." Of course, this was a silly sort of thing, but that's exactly what I thought. The devil with being hopeless! I'm still alive! I'm still breathing, and as long as I'm breathing I may as well do what I can. And at that point that's what I did.

It was at that time that I took a serious look at myself and realized that I could no longer fight for sight, that I had to turn myself around and go in another direction.

In addition to myopia, which I have always had, I was diagnosed with glaucoma, which robs you of your peripheral vision. My low vision turned into "slow vision," and it took about eight years before my "slow vision" turned into practically "no vision." Now once I found out what was happening to me, with a diagnosis of myopia and glaucoma, I realized that I needed to

2

take stock of myself because things were getting serious. Reading was becoming more and more difficult until it was no longer a pleasure. I found that I kept delaying paying my bills, not because I was a miser or didn't have the money, but because it was too hard for me to read the bills and write out the checks. Once I understood that I was now in a new position, I could act on the present particular state of affairs. I said, "Let's see, what can I do? I can stay home in a corner and wait for an aging prince charming to come to me and offer help. But that doesn't seem practical. What else can I do? I can teach. But I'm supposed to be retired. Who's going to give me a job teaching? That seemed out of the question at this point."

It seems silly, but the other thing I knew how to do is go to school. That's what I did. I went back to college and registered for a masters in special education in the low vision section. That's where I learned about myself, what the world of low vision really is, and how to deal with myself and with others who are in this particular kind of physical state.

One thing I learned in college was about being nearsighted. Of course I knew that I had been nearsighted all my life, but I did not know, nor did my family ever realize, that I really, truly was always a low vision person and needed to be treated in a special way to overcome this impairment. The first time anyone recognized that I had less than perfect sight was at about age eight, when an elementary school teacher called my father and said, "I don't believe that Frances is able to see the board from where she's sitting. I believe that she needs glasses." I did get the glasses, and I tried during all my school years to sit in the front of the room so I could see the blackboard. I learned to watch the teacher's hand as she wrote on the blackboard because that would help me decipher what letter she was forming. What I did was "arm read" and "hand read" instead of reading the chalk on the blackboard. I used these clues to get me by.

The second thing I learned is what is meant by impaired vision, in what ways you can deal with impaired vision, and in what ways you can expect eye doctors to deal with it.

The third thing I did was to learn Braille. Although I am not a perfect Braille reader today, nevertheless I have the pleasure of being able to read with my fingers. The world of Braille books is wide and varied. I can read quietly instead of having to be tied to radios, talking books, and TV. Braille may not be the way for you to go. You may not be ready for it. You may never need it. But learning and using Braille is as interesting and as challenging as doing crossword puzzles.

As a result of my courses in low vision education, I turned over stones in my city of San Francisco and found the organizations that help low vision people. From them I took what was good for me, whether it was a discussion group or learning to read Braille or joining a class in ceramics. Just to be with people who were in a similar situation helped me get through the obstacles, until I finally got to where I am now: using my professional expertise not to make money but to set up discussion groups for low vision people and their families and friends so that we can consider, in an upbeat way, the quality of our lives.

That doesn't mean I can do everything all by myself. No, I've lost a part of my independence and I do have to ask people for help. For instance, I can't go around town by myself anymore. I need some kind of help, either an escort or just someone to get me to a particular door. I do need help from people, but as much as I can do myself, I do. I can still give dinner parties. I can make up the menu, I can get the food bought. One or two of my friends might come a little early and help prepare the meal. Then all my friends get together to do the serving and the cleaning up. In a way it makes a better dinner party because everybody's involved. It becomes a cooperative party, and that's my way to have a good social time.

Carpe diem.

These are two words out of old Latin proverbs. ***Carpe*** means "snatch," "grasp at." ***Diem*** means "the day." So the rough translation would be "snatch the day." In other words, catch every moment and use it. A long time ago I went to a support group because I simply felt that I had to be with other people who were experiencing the same distress and despair as I was experiencing, and who also needed to talk about what they were feeling and how they were coping. One of the women in the group had lost her sight very suddenly, from one week practically to the next she was down to no sight to speak of. She had spent a lifetime working in the Post Office, reading addresses all the time, and suddenly she couldn't do it anymore. She, who had been the mainstay of the family, whom everyone had turned to for advice. Well, when she became so badly incapacitated, she was enormously frustrated. She couldn't go to work anymore, couldn't drive, couldn't cook. She was just making a mess of the kitchen. She'd begin to throw pots and pans around, and what is worse, she would snatch up dishes and dash them to the floor. I said, "Kay, that's an awfully expensive indulgence you have. Not only do your dishes cost money, but what are you going to do when you run out of dishes?" It was just her way of expressing her frustration. In my case, I just sat and cried for three days and then finally went out to buy a cappuccino maker. But it took Kay a longer time to get over the anger and the unfairness of what had happened to her before she began to pick up the pieces of her life. Finally, she began to go out and take the long walks that she always loved. She had enough sight to do that. I didn't, I couldn't do that. But everyone to their own capacity, to their own taste, to their own desire. You need to examine what it is in your life that makes you feel good about yourself and then find a way to do it. You may not be able to sew, you may not be able to play golf. But if you think hard enough about it you'll probably find something else to do that will take the place of your once favorite activity.

Kay found out that she needed to ask her family for help. For Kay, and for me, and for lots of other people, learning to ask is a hard come down. We don't want to acknowledge our weakness and we don't want to give up our independence. Unfortunately, the weakness isn't going to go away, and our initial sense of independence needs to become modified so that we can accept the help of kind people graciously. We must always keep in mind that we who need the help must do as much for ourselves as we can. There is nothing quite as easy as making a kind friend into a guilt ridden slave.

Not seeing is more than a frustration or an uncomfortable condition. Indeed, when the loss of sight is serious it is a tragedy because we're missing one of our senses. On the other hand, if you recognize that this tragedy can be overcome, that it's not a terminal illness, then life can go on. I've gone to baseball games, and boy I wish I could see that playing field. I can't, but I can hear the roar of the crowd and smell those hot dogs. I carry a little transistor radio so I can keep up with the plays that I'm not seeing. So I sit down and settle back and enjoy the day, *carpe diem,* for all it's worth.

I propose to show you how you can walk along the streets safely, how you can manage in your own house without going crazy, how you can travel, how you can go to a museum or a movie, whatever it is you want to do. You simply take new and different approaches to habitual activities. Writing this book is an example. I never learned to type. Even if I could type, I couldn't see what I was typing. I don't like to use the talking computers, it's not my cup of tea. So I'm writing this book in an entirely different way. I make notes on one cassette tape recorder. Then I play it onto a second tape, stopping it when I want to add or change something. With a third recorder, I begin to polish what I've said on cassette number one and cassette number two. It's not easy, but if you want to do a thing badly enough, you'll find a way to get it done. Of course, finally I'm going to have to lean on the sighted. Someone will have to reread the manuscript to me and make corrections. In a way it's more interesting because writing is no longer a solitary exercise for me. I turn to another warm body for consultation and reaction to what I'm writing. I find that very pleasant, and always have. When I taught on the university level, as chairman of the department I would have my own secretary. Even when I could see I would throw all of the paperwork on somebody else's desk. I find that I'm still doing the same thing. Whether I'm blind or not, I still like to have a secretary to do all of the shuffling of papers that I never enjoyed doing. These days I enjoy it doubly because my secretary is even more involved with what I'm thinking and doing than ever before. I'm not solitary and I am alone only by my own choice.

Since my sight began to diminish in 1980, I suffered a loss much more serious to me than the loss of sight. My most cherished son died in that period. His loss is a bitter sweetness. He left me his home and his circle of friends, but most important, his greatest legacy, he left his thirteen-year old daughter to me to raise. Believe me, that granddaughter of mine, Christine, has been the carrot before my nose. I had no time to mourn the loss of sight. I had no time really to mourn my son. She and I knew that instead of mourning we would celebrate each day and what each day brings us. So I would have to say that there are tragedies that touch us even more deeply than changing sight. My daughter Amy said to me, "Mother, how lucky you are." Now, this in the face of a death and loss of sight! She said, "How lucky you are. You have a second chance to raise a thirteen-year-old." We laughed at that because in my experience and in her experience a thirteen-year old female is something else again to deal with. Christine survived, and I survived. It wasn't easy, but whoever promised me a rose garden? My life was mine to cultivate, with or without watering, with or without compost, but on the other hand one can pluck the flowers and enjoy their bloom and their aroma. Life is *dancing in the dark.* Maybe it's two steps forward and one step back, but you do progress.

And so my life became one of acceptance and invention. Acceptance of the condition. Invention of ways to circumvent it. In my case the serious change of eyesight occurred with age. That is, by the time I was about sixty Mother Nature was dealing me the hand that she had kept ready for me throughout the years. Through a professional career, through a marriage, through raising two children, through a perfectly satisfying social life, poor eyesight never deterred me. I had always suspected that people saw colors and sunshine and light in much more of a blaze than I did, but I have always accepted the condition of my vision. Even now, when I've got nothing more than some peripheral light and dark that tells me whether it's daylight or nighttime or whether there's an electric light on or not, I simply accept it–because this is the way it's supposed to be for me and there's nothing I can do about it. So I bend with the blow. I don't fight it, I join it. That's the message this book contains: how to stop the fight and get on with life.

In the following pages I will share with you some of my experiences in the hope that you can match them to your needs. The main point is that you will need to turn yourself around in your own way, at your own time, at your own speed, and within the limits of your self-love. You must not hate yourself for what you don't have, but love yourself for what you do have. Mourning, moping, and complaining may be necessary for a while but ultimately will get you nowhere. Courage and laughter, on the other hand, will take you a long way on your route to a happy, satisfying existence. You'd be surprised at how many strokes you get from folks because they are amazed at what you can do in spite of not seeing. You must drop the psychology of sight and pick up the psychology of non sight.

Think of yourself as an explorer. You set out to find a spice route to India, to find you have instead discovered another world. "Hey, I need help to explore this new world," you say.

You need to explore a new world, find out what it's all about, and then to strike out into it to make it work for you. So we are all explorers. Our new destination can often be quite exotic. Think of that. It's exotic because it's quite different from the expected, from the norm.

I'm quite apt to ask a friend who comes to visit me in the late afternoon and into the evening to turn on the light. I don't necessarily need to have the light on for myself. I say, "Oh, you poor thing. Find the light switch. I'm so sorry for you that you need light to get around." Or, a friend of mine is looking for something in a drawer and can't find it. I say, "Just a minute. Let me go through that drawer." I feel through and in no time flat I have the object, whatever it is. I say, "You poor thing. All you can do is see. You don't know what it means to feel for a thing. Fingers, you see, need to be as educated as mine are."

With courage and laughter our circle of friends is enlarged. We're not replacing our circle of friends, we're enlarging them. We include people with whom we have specialized interests in common. With the commonality of interests with these new friends you also have the opportunity to laugh at your failures, your foibles, your frustrations, which you can't do with people who have sight. In other words, in a group of people who are visually impaired, at least you can laugh at yourself safely. The slogan here might be *Go, but go slow.*

I have found that I have developed certain capacities that I never thought I had. For instance, in talking to sighted people, I found that I had to slow down, to take the time necessary to explain what it is I needed. I couldn't be grouchy or grumpy or complaining about it either. In addition, I needed the patience to wait until a friend was ready to help me. One day I was sitting with a group of people in the chambers of the city board of supervisors. We were waiting for a certain bit of legislation to come to discussion. There were about eight of us, sitting there quietly. All of us had low vision, to one degree or another. Some could see the people who were in the front of the room. A woman next to me who had no sight at all, and never had, was sitting there knitting. With us there was a sighted guide, a woman who had brought us there because negotiating the steps and elevators at city hall was a bit too much for us. She said to me that she always had been aware how patient sight-impaired people are.

That impressed me. Through the years I've always remembered the word that she used, "patience." Taking it easy. It will get done, not in this instant, but in a little while. On the other hand, I can get quite nervous if I'm waiting at a ticket counter or at the airport until somebody takes my ticket and takes care of me because I'm not sure whether they've forgotten me or not. Nevertheless, as much as I feel like screaming, I don't. I simply wait. If things got really tough for me I might ask a polite question to someone I imagine is behind the counter, "Are you there," I'd say, holding my white cane up in an obvious position. "Are you there? I need to ask you a question?" Just like that and no other way, without any querulous tone at all, because you can catch more flies with honey than you can with vinegar.

Chapter 2
BETWEEN YOU AND YOUR DOCTOR

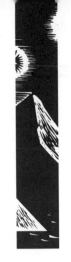

As soon as you notice a change in your vision you need to have a consultation with an ophthalmologist. If you don't have an ophthalmologist, you can ask your primary care doctor to recommend one. You can also get a referral to an ophthalmologist from the American Academy of Ophthalmologists or from a local hospital eye clinic. Sometimes your friends may recommend an ophthalmologist, saying, "He or she is the best one." However, he or she may not be the best one for you. Later in this chapter, I'll talk about what to look for when you choose a doctor.

You might choose to consult with an optometrist. An optometrist is trained to prescribe and grind lenses for eyeglasses and contact lenses, as well as to suggest adaptive appliances for better vision. An ophthalmologist, however, will be concerned with your entire medical history as well. Your eyes are part of your body and may be affected by diseases and conditions that you may not ordinarily associate with eye disorders.

Your ophthalmologist will use a variety of instruments to examine your eyes. Dr. William Good, Assistant Professor of Ophthalmology at The University of California in San Francisco (UCSF) specifies the following as basic tools of the trade:

1. **Ophthalmoscope.** This is a light source that provides some magnification and enables the ophthalmologist to check the optic nerve and retina.

2. **Indirect Ophthalmoscope.** This is a funny-looking hat with a light source that the ophthalmologist wears on the forehead. Using a 30- or 40-Diopter lens magnifier held in front of the patient's eye, the ophthalmologist can examine the entire retina.

3. **Slit Lamp.** This is a magnifying gadget that enables the ophthalmologist to look at the front surface of the eye (e.g.,the cornea or the eyelids.)

4. **Phoropter.** These are crazy-looking goggles with lenses in them. The patient puts on the phoropter so the ophthalmologist can measure the patient for glasses.

5. **Retinoscope.** This instrument looks a little like an ophthalmoscope. It provides the light that enables ophthalmologists to check for refractive errors (near-sightedness) without necessarily having to use the phoropter.

6. **Tonometer.** This instrument is used to check for glaucoma. It has a blue light and a cone-shaped device that presses the surface of the cornea to measure the intraocular pressure.

After your eye exam your ophthalmologist will tell you what is going on. You hope it's good news, but sometimes it's not so good. In fact, your ophthalmologist may be the bearer of very unpleasant news. Of course, you will be devastated if your ophthalmologist tells you that very little can be done to restore your vision. One woman described her sudden loss of vision and the shocking news from her ophthalmologist as follows: "One afternoon at the end of my work day, I found that I couldn't read the papers I needed to file. I thought it was because I hadn't turned the lights on in the office. When I came to work the next morning it was still the same story. In the bright morning light I wasn't able to read. By 1:00 P.M. I was in the ophthalmologist's office. By 3:00 P.M. he told me I would be blind within two months. By 5:00 P.M. I went home and wanted to commit suicide. I lost my job, I had to give up driving, and I lost my position of leadership in my family. But in the end, I gained my family's loving cooperation, and I learned a way of coping with sight loss that has added to my spiritual strength."

Like this woman, at the moment you hear bad news about your vision you may feel that life is over. You might feel so angry you want to scream, or so sad and upset that you can't hold back the tears. Or you might feel frightened. "When my doctor told me I was going blind," another person told me, "I stopped going downtown. I stopped my daily walks. I stopped visits to the farmer's market. I stopped everything but breathing. I stayed home in bed. It took two years for my friends to pull me out of the doldrums." It is perfectly natural to feel hopeless and overwhelmed when you first get a diagnosis of vision loss.

Unfortunately, your ophthalmologist might not have the time to give you the emotional support you need. Ask him to refer you to an agency serving the visually impaired. These agencies have social workers, counselors, and support groups to help you cope with the emotional distress and other unpleasant consequences of vision loss and to help you adjust to a new way of life. You might also want to contact a low vision clinic at a nearby university hospital to find out if they are familiar with any special treatments for your condition.

You can learn to live your life in new and different ways. You can learn a new way to manage food preparation, how to use a cane, how to market for groceries. You can learn what to do when you feel depressed or scared. You can learn to effectively use partial sight.

It is important that you actively participate in planning what you will do. You have the ultimate power and authority for the decisions you make about how to conduct your life. It is important not to put yourself down. Instead, you need to be good to yourself and find things you can still enjoy. It is to your advantage to be open to finding new interests and to learning new ways to live your life, inside and outside your home. In the chapters ahead I'll share with you some of the things I've learned that have worked for me.

Here are two anecdotes that have a common thread. The common thread is anxiety, sudden changes in sight, doctor's diagnoses, ignorance of the condition that caused your sight loss, hopelessness and despair, and finally getting on with one's life even without sufficient professional support.

"When I was a young man of thirty-five, a productive business person, I was driving along one day and noticed that I wasn't keeping the car on the straight and narrow, I was either hitting the side of the road to the right or hitting the island to the left. It's lucky I didn't kill myself or anybody else. I went to an eye doctor. He said, 'I don't know what's wrong with you. We'll have to wait and see.' So we waited, and as we waited I went blind. I had some peripheral vision to the right and to the left, but no vision ahead. I couldn't read. That was the end, I thought, of my career. And to a large degree it was. I never found out what it was that caused this sudden onset of almost, but not quite, total blindness. I can see light, I can see out of the corners of my eyes. I can even read that way, but surely not good enough for me to read leases and legal papers having to do with the insurance business. I didn't have anyone to talk to. I fretted it out and at age thirty-five, in the prime of my life, I needed to start all over again. I did it on my own, with no support from any doctor and no encouragement."

"At about the age of forty I discovered that I wasn't seeing as well as I used to. I went to the doctor and he said, 'Well, you have retinitis pigmentosa, and this kind of condition means that you'll be losing sight as you go along in life. If Mother Nature is kind to you, you'll have the sight that you have now, and if Mother Nature is not kind, little by little, the lights will go out.' So I went home and decided to give up everything: my job, my life as a professional, my social life, the happiness and laughter, the sociability that I was used to, and go sit in a corner and just plain die. And, of course, feeling bad as I did, I walked around complaining to myself, Why me, God? But that didn't get me anywhere. So eventually I went to the doctor. I went to an eye clinic and said to the doctor, 'Why do I see these funny lights at the sides of my eyes and these rings inside my eyeballs?' Later on I discovered that Van Gogh had the same condition. I continued, 'Why is this happening? What does it mean?' And he said, 'I'll have to examine you to find out exactly what your condition is.' So he took all sorts of tests. Then he said, 'Well, that's glaucoma. It could be arrested. You'll have to find out with medication.' I said to him, 'Well, in addition to that, I see this haze. What's going to happen?' He said, 'It's going to get worse.' No support, no comfort, no pity, no empathy, just, 'Your eyesight is going to get worse.' He never explained at all what the blur was and why I had it."

Now what do these people have in common? Both had diminished vision of one sort or another. They both went to doctors. They both received diagnoses and reports that were discouraging and negative, with no hope for regaining sight. They meekly accepted what their physician said. They were out of hope and out of fight. Out of the strength to sit there and ask the doctor questions, questions, and more questions. Of course, in all fairness to these people, it's true that asking a question about something you know nothing or very little about is difficult. Even in a classroom you can't ask your teacher a question unless you have a glimmer of what the teacher is talking about. The same thing goes for the doctor's office. The lesson to be learned here is that you don't rush out of the office. You sit there and say, "doctor, please take a little more time with me to explain why this has happened to me, what it means. Can you explain it to me in terms of the physiology of the eye? Can you explain it to me in terms of how I can get on with my life; can you give me insight or hope or encouragement? How can I handle this turn around of circumstances?" It's the obligation of the physician to have empathy and a bedside manner. But you, the patient, also have an obligation. It is up to you to ask questions and not be afraid to take up the doctor's time. It's up to you to be brave enough to say, "I don't understand what you're saying. Can you break it down a little more for me so that I can understand?" If you can't elicit the response you need from the doctor you're dealing with, then find another one because your life is at stake.

Dr. James Tulsky, whose special area of interest is medical ethics, spoke at a forum sponsored by the University of California San Francisco's Department of Ophthalmology. The attendees were all low vision people. "I want to consider the question of patients talking to doctors," he said. "I believe that this is where the largest breakdown in understanding between physician and patient occurs. No matter what the issue, whether it's death or dying, durable power of attorney, living wills, or

16

physical conditions including eyesight, the doctor should be ready and willing to talk to you at your level of understanding, usually without medical jargon. Doctors are usually willing to talk about these things, but sometimes they're uncomfortable about bringing bad news. After all, doctors are human beings also. But of course you, the patient, are a person too, and you need to speak up and say what's on your mind, what's in your heart, and how you understand your situation. You need to ask questions, even though they may seem obvious and silly. If you don't ask, you'll never know. You may get the impression that the doctor is angry with you or impatient to get you out of the office. But remember, you are the person who is at risk and you are the subject at hand, you are the patient and you are entitled not only to receive help from this person as a physician, but also to receive support and bolster your shaky ego. You may think it's hard to ask questions about a topic about which you know very little. Yet you actually know more then you think. You know how you feel now, you know how you see now. You know how you used to feel, you know how you used to see. So, on the basis of your own experiences, you can ask questions."

Dr. Tulsky went on to talk about choosing a doctor who is right for you. "It is always best," he said, "to start with a primary care doctor, often a general internist, before you go on to a specialist. He or she can help you choose a specialist for your condition." But what if you find an ophthalmologist, for instance, who is used to dealing with eyes but not the person behind the eyes? Dr. Tulsky knows that many people leave their physician's offices feeling frustrated. The physician has been too hurried and they haven't had enough questions answered. It's clear that some practitioners are better than others in talking to patients as people. After all, your physician is as human as you are, with his or her own strengths and failings. But if you're not satisfied, it's time to move on to another doctor.

Interviewing physicians may seem like a novel idea, and of course these first consultations cost money. These are large expenses. Make sure that your primary and secondary insurance carriers cover the cost of ophthalmological examinations. But remember that with whomever you choose you will be establishing a long term relationship, through months and maybe even years—so be frank and tell him the kind of doctor you're looking for. Then he can tell you if he fits the bill not only as a professional person with a diploma, but also as a person with whom you can speak heart-to-heart. It's a match of expertise as well as personality.

Here's a checklist of your considerations:

1. Is this person relaxed enough with you to answer your questions?

2. Does this person speak clearly and in understandable English? Do you understand his vocabulary?

3. Is this a person with whom you can feel comfortable?

4. Is this a person with whom you can speak about your difficult daily problems in readjustment?

5. Does he or she explain to you the progress of your eye impairment?

6 Has he or she told you what resources there are in your community for further help?

7. Is the doctor's office close enough for you to get to without too much trouble?

8. What are the doctor's fees? Will it be adjusted for you?

Shopping around isn't easy no matter how you do it, but it is important. Let's hope you have health insurance to cover your needs.

When you walk into a doctor's office armed with a series of questions, you'll quickly learn to find out how much cooperation you will get from this physician over and above medical knowledge. No doctor, says Dr. Tulsky, will think the less of you for persisting in your drive for information, not only about your eye condition but also about the pharmaceuticals he's prescribing for you, for example, and their possible side effects. Dr. Tulsky said, "A doctor's respect for you will rise if you are interested in learning more about your condition."

Good questions get good answers. For instance, if you say to your ophthalmologist, "What is the true prognosis of my condition?" he must turn around and face you to tell you the truth. It may be harsh, unsettling, and even devastating, but nevertheless you will know the truth because you asked the question. You might ask: "What are the chances of saving whatever sight I have?" "Are there any agencies to which I can turn to help me adjust to my present condition?" "What sources are there in my community for helping low vision people?" These questions can open the way to a real exchange. That's the difference between a doctor flat-out saying, "You're going to go blind in three months," discussion over, and your settling down to have a conversation in which you can begin to understand why this is happening.

Dr. Tulsky told his audience: "When you go to your doctor, have your questions written down. Bring a friend or family member with you to listen to the answers. Two heads are better than one." If you don't have a friend or family member to go along with you, you might get a volunteer from one of the local community agencies. Dr. Tulsky went on: "And bring a tape recorder as well. Of course, ask the doctor's permission to use that tape recorder so you can go home and review everything he said." In fact, if you get to the point where you can't write down your questions, consider putting your questions on tape. You've opened up a two-way street toward a satisfying and informative visit. If you hand the doctor a list of questions or a tape of your questions, he begins at least to turn to you as a person. The doctor can understand your concerns and try to help you with them, while you start getting your issues resolved. When we hear bad news we tend to be so upset that we forget that we have questions. But if you put the question list on the doctor's desk then you don't have to worry about remembering.

Here are some essential questions you will probably want to ask:

1. What is the nature of my condition?
2. What medications are you prescribing? What do they do?
3. How often do I take them?
4. Do they have side effects?
5. If they do have side effects, what should I do about them?
6. Should I call you any time I have a pain or some sudden change in my sight?

If you find that your doctor is waffling through these questions, then it's time to look for another ophthalmologist. Or, at the least, it's time to get a second opinion. Good communication leads to good understanding. Good understanding leads to relaxation of your anxiety. It may not relieve all your anxiety, but understanding will help you get your life reordered, so that even though you're functioning on a different level, you are indeed functioning.

In general, negotiating the health care system can be incredibly difficult. Dr. Tulsky says that even for him, as a physician, it can often be difficult to match a patient with an appropriate physician. Recommendations may come to you from a social worker, a friend, another physician, your next-door neighbor. These are people with whom you're speaking in confidence on a friendly or semi-professional level. However, a casual thought such as, "Oh, he's a wonderful doctor," may lead you astray. You need some hard facts when choosing a doctor. You may expect every doctor to be technically competent, but not every one will be a good match for you. Seek and ye shall find; *remember patience.*

Chapter 3
ORGANIZING YOUR PERSONAL LIFE

As a sighted person you have organized your house in your own way. When problems arise with the gradual diminishing of your sight you naturally make adjustments and changes. But to a large extent, even as your sight is changing, you can keep your house as it is.

Moving around the house, however, is something of a new matter now. Obviously, you need to be more cautious. But caution is not enough. You need to organize so you can remember where everything is. You need to get into the habit of returning everything to its place so you can find it next time. When I first became a low vision person my mind felt full of cotton wool, my ears and my brain seemed stuffed, and nothing seemed to work. But little by little, as I applied myself to living a self-respecting life under new conditions, I developed skills and methods that enabled me to live in a way which, if not perfect, is in some ways better than before. One of the most important skills I developed was remembering. Remembering locations of things is a key to coming out of chaos and restoring calm.

The best aid to memory is organization. There are endless ways to organize your house so that you can find things easily. For example, if you have difficulty with cans or jars, one piece of attached tape might identify the tomato sauce, while two attached pieces indicate the tomato paste. There are many appliances, manuals, catalogs, hardware, and other aids for organization. You don't have to follow anyone else's ideas though they may be good jumping-off places. You might read in one manual, for instance, that white coffee cups are good because you can see more easily where the coffee level is when you pour. But, as is true for me, if you can't see that well you've got to find another way. I've learned to judge how full the coffee cup is by the weight of it. You might try that, or you may have to find yet another method. It's a process of discovering, testing, and rediscovering what works for you in your situation. But in the end it's your situation, your life. All the suggestions of other people, including me, are only that, suggestions. As I like to say, even to myself, "You have to turn over your own stones." There's no way to avoid doing personal research with all its trial and error. You have to find your own way of moving from chaos to calm! For example, I used to try to remember what my few medicines were by shape and size. I don't bother anymore. I simply put one kind over to the left in the medicine cabinet, another over to the right, another on a lower shelf, and so on. But maybe you'll want to mark yours with masking tape, Scotch tape, or a rubber band. Another example: I know a man who only buys socks of one color so he never has to worry about separating and matching pairs. But the same man likes to hàve many different colored ties. So, on one hanger he keeps gray ties, on another brown, on another patterns with a red cast, and so on. That's a method that works for him.

Clearly, there are infinite possible variations. I separate my underwear in plastic bags by type: pantyhose, panties, bras, and so on. I hang certain skirts and blouses of matching colors on the same hangers. Other blouses I hang separately because I can tell the colors by the feel of their material and style. But one could easily imagine other systems: a marker inside the collar;

or a marker on the hangers—say a little plastic letter (B for blue, for example).

You can gather helpful gadgets for these purposes from catalogs, by visiting stores that sell equipment for the blind, or just by visiting hardware stores or other shops that sell organizing gimmicks for closets. You don't have to buy right away. You can look and think and gather ideas for your own situation. In San Francisco, for instance, there's a store called Hold Everything that carries devices for storage for every room in the home. If you go when they're not busy you can get many ideas. Of course, no system is perfect. Just like any sighted person, you will lose things in your home. Don't drive yourself crazy. If you can't find it after a while, forget it. You'll have to replace it. Adjusting to blindness is often a question of substituting one thing in your life for another, and letting go when nothing else will do.

There are lots of little tricks that a low vision person can use to make everyday life less difficult, but they take a long time to fall into place. Over the months and years, if you give yourself patience and love, you'll learn all you need to know and your life will become easier and richer.

All of these methods, systems, and tricks, by the way, are technically known as *independent living skills.* One caveat: Many of the books on this subject are written by sighted people and the suggestions don't always work in every detail for people without sight, another reason to create your own ways.

Having stressed the importance of using your own methods and ingenuity, let me give you some ideas. I'll discuss some important aspects of daily living with blindness that may help you understand what's involved in living in your house in a new way. This is what worked for me, room by room, in my house.

THE KITCHEN

The first rule in the kitchen is to know what's there by making an inventory of your supplies and organizing everything for your convenience. One reason this is so important is that you will probably have other people coming into your kitchen and working, and you'll need to be able to direct them (constantly) where to find and put things. So give everything a place and return everything to its place. This rule holds for cupboards, closets, and the refrigerator.

In order to do this you will have to keep your memory active. I'm constantly feeling around and keeping track of things and putting them back in their places. If someone brings groceries for me, I generally won't let that person put them away. I put them away myself, according to my system, so I know I can find them. It is absolutely routine, however, for my friends to make themselves a cup of tea and forget to put the cup in the sink afterward or the milk carton back in the refrigerator.

Which brings me to the second important rule of operation. Be sure and tell your visitors to put things back exactly where they found them. You may feel shy about this at first, but if you don't you're in for trouble. For instance, my dear granddaughter, having lived with me for years, knows that everything has its place. However, she'll come back from college for a week-and-a-half and afterward I go crazy because I can't find that special can opener of mine. I search everywhere and don't know if it's still here or if she took it back to college with her. Even with all my experience, I still fail to insist enough that people return things to their place. So if people work in your kitchen for you, tell them, over and over, as often as necessary, to put things back. It's hard playing nag like this so do it with a smile, but do it. It's crucial if you don't want your life to descend into chaos after you have organized it.

ESTABLISHING A SYSTEM

You can systematize what's in the kitchen in many ways. At first you may need someone to identify things for you, read labels on cans, and so forth. Gradually you develop a way of identifying things. There are many tricks. For instance, one way I help myself keep track of food supplies is to leave them in the plastic bags they came in rather than putting them in standardized containers that won't tell me anything about what's inside. I can feel the plastic bags and pretty well tell what's in them, such as raisins or flour.

KITCHEN SAFETY

In order to be safe I try to shun as many electrical appliances as possible: mixers, for instance, or juicers and electric can openers. You can get quite a lot of these gadgets in battery-operated cordless models and I recommend them everywhere in the home. Avoiding wires is a way of avoiding shocks and confusion in general.

For the same reason, wherever I have an opportunity I have electricians install outlets, especially at counter level so I can avoid a confusing spaghetti of wires. Consider the alternative. I need to attach a radio and have no available outlet. So I'm on the floor, crawling, tracking down an extension cord with a multiple head. Eventually I find the extension cord, and then I keep crawling until I finally find the head of the cord with the multiple outlets. At this point I plug the radio into a cord head. Then, holding on so I won't lose it (my eyes are in my hands at this point in my life), I have to reach up and turn on the radio. Sure enough, it doesn't work. Well, you can get an idea of how complicated it all is. I leave the radio turned on, but now I have to trace the extension cord back to the baseboard. Still crawling on the floor blind, mind you, behind furniture, groping to find the baseboard outlet and trying not to get a shock in the process, eventually I discover that the extension cord was not firmly plugged in. It is with this sort of incident in mind that I say go to batteries and as many wall outlets as you can afford.

For safety's sake I have become a fan of microwave cooking. There's no danger of leaving gas or electric burners on or burning yourself on an electric coil that takes a long time to cool down. You'll probably want to keep a gas or electric range for certain uses, but get a microwave oven with a few buttons that can be marked for you. Have someone read a microwave cookbook to you, or even better have it read onto a tape. You'll have to listen to it over and over. But it's worth it. Microwave cooking is very precise; you get sure control. You can learn to cook almost everything this way. You can also get the same safe use out of a toaster oven or an electric fry pan.

Some other safety tips: Keep sharp knives all together in a safe place (but you probably did that anyway before you lost your sight). Keep your cabinets closed so you don't bang into them. Check to see that the burners on your stove are turned off, and the faucets also. Some of this I can do just by listening. *Remember: don't put it off, turn it off.*

THE COMMAND STATION

In my kitchen I have a little comfort command station fitted with a comfortable chair, a low table for the phone, my "memo pad," tape recorder, a radio, and of course a clock. Clocks in my house are of two kinds: those for my sighted visitors and those for me. The first are conventional clocks. The second are clocks that "talk" in one way or another. There are an enormous variety of such talking clocks on the market. There are those that actually speak the hour and the minute when you press the button, those that chime the quarter-hours, those that chime the hour and minute when you press a lever, and so on. I love gadgets, so I have all of these and more. I keep only one on the table near my kitchen easy chair. I also have room for a cup and a small dish. You want to have spots throughout the house where you can sit or lie comfortably and be organized to do several things: phone, make memos, drink, eat, tell time, and so on. These are also my command comfort stations.

NEW COOKING TECHNIQUES

Not only will you have to organize your kitchen things, you will have to learn to use them in new ways. Pouring liquids and cutting foods are two areas where you may need some new techniques.

If you need a cup of cold liquid, milk, water, whatever, pour it over a bowl in the sink. If you should overpour or aim incorrectly, the overflow will go into the bowl.

Hot liquids are another matter. If you need to measure out a cup of something hot, pour the liquid cold into your measuring cup and then pour it into your pot to heat up. That way, when the liquid is hot, you have the exact quantity you need. This method is safer than starting with a larger quantity of hot liquid and then trying to measure the amount you need.

To measure oil it is handy to keep it in a wide-mouthed jar in your refrigerator. It will pour more slowly than oil at room temperature, enabling you to better control the pouring of a small amount. I learned this, by the way, from a chef who went blind. He also taught me to bend a teaspoon or tablespoon so that the bowl faces up, like a tiny ladle. Then, when you want a teaspoon or tablespoon of a liquid, you just dip the bent spoon in and pull up slowly. Using a funnel is also a handy way of controlling liquids.

Cutting has only one rule: cut the food, not your fingers. A useful tip for this is to get in the habit of folding your fingers into your hand so that when the knife comes down it slices past your knuckles and not into your exposed fingers.

As for cooking in general, try to keep things simple. One big help is using foolproof simple recipes. The ideal recipe is one in which you can dump all the ingredients into a single pot and forget about it. Let me give you some examples of this approach.

If you want to make a pot roast you can skip all the old-fashioned recipes and use this one. Put a layer of sliced onions at the bottom of a pot or, to make things even simpler, just throw in some whole small cooking onions. Next put in the meat. Dump your vegetables on top, any you wish, all your old refrigerator remains like soft celery and carrots, mushrooms, potatoes cut or not, and so on. Then, secret number one, pour in a can of beer. If you want to thicken the juice, save some of the beer, stir some flour into it, and then throw that in. The next step is very interesting (a chef friend's secret). Make a little paste out of flour and water and rub it around the rim of the pot so that when you put the lid on it really sticks tight. Put the whole thing in the oven at 350 degrees and cook it for about fifteen minutes per pound of meat. That's it, and if you don't like it, let me know!

Here's another very simple recipe: "Hopple-Popple." It's scrambled eggs with anything you want to put in, from green pepper to onions to potatoes.

What quick recipes do you know? What recipes do your friends know? It doesn't take much searching, and there are many cookbooks that can help, to put together an interesting repertoire of easy-to-cook dishes.

THE LIVING ROOM

Although I spend a lot of time at my comfort station in the kitchen, the living room is really my center of operations. It has a desk in it that often gets piled up with letters and papers and all sorts of junk. My once-a-week reader comes and, in her wisdom and patience, untangles my web. Following the general rule of keeping things organized, I have a pretty good idea of where everything is: the checkbook and the extra checks, pens, paper clips, forms for my health insurance, and so on. I don't use these things myself, but I know where they are. This allows me to tell sighted people where to find things I may need their help with.

In my living room I also have a rocking chair. I like the rocking chair very much because, in various ways, it is a source of comfort many times during the day. On a little table beside it, like the one next to my kitchen chair, I have a telephone, a small portable radio, a tape recorder which is my memo pad, and the controls for my television. All of this is easily accessible.

You may well ask what I'm doing with a television. I'm interested in all sorts of programs, nature, theater, and news. Even though I can't see, I still can get a lot out of these programs. In the documentary programs I can listen to the descriptions, and in the dramatic shows, I supply through my imagination what I don't see. Obviously I miss the visual enjoyment of a period piece on *Masterpiece Theatre*, for example, but with interview shows, of which there are so very many, I do very well. Certain soap operas or situation comedies I also enjoy tremendously.

"Audiovision" is available now for blind people. It's a device you hook up to your television that plugs into one channel of your stereo system. Some programs on television are accompanied by audio descriptions that are specially designed for blind people. Some states offer more of this than others and you will have to call your local television stations to find out what's available by way of audio description.

The couch in my living room is where I assume my executive position, flat out. I have an afghan for extra comfort, a pillow, my radio on a nearby table, and I must confess, all around it are crumbs from snacks I've eaten. To keep the person who helps with the cleaning from going mad and killing me, I have a scatter rug to gather the debris of crumbs lest they get rubbed irrevocably into the carpet. Here on the couch I lie and listen to the television and the radio, and also read my Braille book. In this room the one item that has a long cord is the telephone, so that I can move from the rocking chair to the couch and still have the phone handy. But this one long cord is arranged in such a way as to avoid the traffic pattern into and out of the room, to prevent anyone's tripping over it, especially me. I do have to make a special effort to remember where the cord is.

I listen to a wonderful radio service that exists for the print impaired. It's called *In Touch* and is broadcast nationally by satellite. Here I find, twenty-four hours a day, readings of newspapers and magazines: *The New York Times,* for instance or *The Wall Street Journal,* or *Playboy,* and so on. Anytime I turn on the radio somebody is reading to me. There are also children's programs, a book-of-the week, local sports, computer news, interviews with local personalities, and so on. You need to have a special radio to pick up this service, and you can get it free. If you call *In-Touch* in New York City, they will give you the number of your local service. It's a great service, useful and comforting. In fact I had a program of my own on a local station, which I did with two sighted people, called *Cabbages and Kings.* We talked about performing arts events, travel, dining out, and even gave recipes for eating in, always with special reference to the blind. In reviewing restaurants, for example, we gave special tips for blind people about how to get there and how to manage once you are there.

THE BATHROOM

The essential thing in the bathroom, as everywhere else in the house, is organization and keeping things in place. That means, for example, that before you turn on the spigots you know exactly where everything is that you will need to use with the water: soap, toothbrush, toothpaste, washcloth, shaving cream, towels, and so on. It also means learning to know your environment all over again from the perspective of your other senses. How many times, for example, have I run a bath and only later realized that I had forgotten to check the plug with my hands to make sure that it was in firmly and correctly. Hearing is also important. Like it or not, when I enter the bathroom or pass by I will listen to make sure there's no water running in the wrong places. Is the toilet-tank water quiet? Is there water gurgling, dripping, or running from the shower?

In arranging your bathroom it's important to recognize that you are more liable to slip than a sighted person and that you need to take measures to prevent that. Carpeting can be a good idea. Or you can buy special non-skid tiles for covering a bathroom floor. Non-skid rubber mats in the shower and next to the shower are also very helpful. There are also similarly prepared non-skid surfaces for the bottom of a shower stall to use in addition to any mat you put down. Another important safety measure is to keep oils, including bath oils, off the shower floor.

I keep a walker in the shower to balance myself. It's a good idea, also, to arrange for grab bars to be installed in obvious places such as near the toilet or anywhere else where you might get up and down or reach, and therefore be liable to slip. Towel bars, if they are strong and firmly fixed to the wall, can also serve as grab bars. However, if you intend to use them for this purpose in an unfamiliar house or a hotel room, test them first.

In fact, using any bathroom except my own always presents a problem and a challenge. The problem is safety, and the challenge is figuring out where everything is and how I can use what I need without harm. Obviously, I will already have mastered the challenges of my own bathroom at home. They include finding the handle of the toilet flush, finding out how the spigots operate, where the handles are, which way they turn on and off, how the water strikes the bottom of the basin, how open I can have the spigots without drenching the whole room with ricocheting spray from thundering faucets, how the stopper operates to open and close, and so on.

The major test in the bathroom, whether at home or elsewhere, is taking a shower. Before you turn on the water in that shower you need to find out how the stopper operates so you can have it open. And you have to know how to operate the faucets safely so that you can get the temperature you want and not scald yourself. Adjust the water temperature before you actually get into the shower. Before you even do that, find out how the shower curtain or door works, whether there's a bar to grab onto or, if there is none, how you can support yourself against a wall as you are getting in and out. You should also examine the floor of the shower stall or tub with your hands to make sure the surface isn't slippery. If it is, you'll need to arrange for a mat or towel to be put there to help you stand securely.

You've got to be prepared and cautious. Lack of caution in a strange bathroom can mean catastrophe. I was visiting a friend in his house and was about to take a shower when suddenly the fellow entered. "What are you doing here?" I cried, going on to insist on my privacy. "I'm very sorry," he answered, "but I was nervous about your hurting yourself with scalding water." I, armed with my watchwords *preparation* and *caution,* was equipped to deal with this perilous situation, both the scalding water and, therefore, his unwanted presence. "I asked you and you showed me how the faucets operate," I reassured him. "Thank you kindly for your attention," I continued, "you can relax, I can take care of myself." He left, and I was quite pleased.

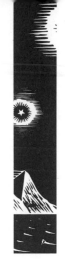

Chapter 4
COMMUNICATING

READING

Just because you have low vision doesn't mean you have to give up your favorite authors. A fair amount of your "reading" can come over the radio through the special stations for the blind. You can learn Braille, too. You can also get various gadgets from local libraries that will help you to read. Some libraries offer machines that enlarge printed books for those with low vision. Some have machines that translate written books into sound. Some have cassette recorders for "talking books," of which there are more and more nowadays. There are also record players on which you can listen to books.

Braille, of course, is slower than the reading you're accustomed to. Not only does Braille take a long time to learn but you read it at about one-third the speed of reading with vision. For these reasons, and others, the world of the blind is slow. But if you are blind, it is precisely time that you're likely to have a lot of, which allows you to learn that essential quality the blind must have: patience. Patience is not such a bad thing to master for any human being, sighted or blind.

READERS

A "reader" is any person who helps you read something. This can be a friend who happens to be with you when you pick up your mail at the front door and whom you ask to read the return addresses. A reader can also be someone who gives you secretarial assistance on a regular basis or someone who reads whole books to you.

People willing to make themselves regularly available as readers are hard to come by, but they are worth their weight in gold, so it's good to make an effort to find one, or more likely, a succession of people over time. For a successful union you have to understand each other's needs and capacities. If you find someone who suits you, cherish it as a match made in heaven.

Most readers are volunteers: college students, retired people, high school kids, kind neighbors. To find someone, apply to community organizations, or try advertising. You can advertise in a local paper or a community center bulletin board. It's not easy to find someone who is willing to be a consistent and patient pair of eyes for you. Sometimes you can find a person who will do it for pay. With any reader, paid or not, be prepared to go to extra lengths to be courteous and generous, just as with all the people who help you in one way or another. Anyone who performs these services for the blind is doing a real service, and on behalf of blind people everywhere I want to thank you. We need you. There are never enough readers for the blind, every blind person can use more help with reading.

WRITING TECHNIQUES

I don't write Braille particularly well. I learned it late in life and it takes a lot of practice to become proficient at writing. I like to take a little portable Braille typewriter along when I'm on a trip or a weekend visit with friends. In this way I can use the time when my friends are out shopping to do my own studying or systematic reflection or note taking.

As for writing with a pen, I usually print, but often people say they can't read it. My writing was never terribly legible in the first place, and it's even worse now. So when I need to do essential writing I employ two methods. I have a paid or volunteer person write for me, especially checks, a reliable person who knows how to balance the checkbook accurately. The second method I use is with a tape recorder. A tape recorder is especially handy, not only for dictating material that may later be transcribed, but for writing letters, you simply mail the cassette itself. Of course, you need to have the packet in which you put it addressed by someone who can see, but you can slip a tape into an envelope designed for that purpose.

Writing can be hell, especially if you're doing it for publication. You're so dependent on other people, and often on many other people. You can't read what others write, you can't read what you write. You need someone to do your library research for you, write it up, type it and bring it to you. Then you need a reader to read it to you and to help you make your changes and additions. Then back to the typist, then to someone who proofreads it for you, then back to the typist again. And so forth. You get the idea: not only are you dependent on many other personalities, but there are also frustrating time lags between all these stages of the process. As a consequence, because you can't see, you are often not so much writing as supervising, as it were, and at a distance. For all these reasons everything takes much longer than if you were sighted, perhaps three or four times as long.

So here is another place where, as a blind person, you have to exercise patience. Of course, if you are a billionaire and can afford lots of secretaries and editors and overseers it is somewhat simpler. But even then the process is still quite complicated. On the other hand I'm not the only blind person who has managed to write numerous articles, some pamphlets, and now even a book. *Persistence, patience, and organization,* here as in other areas of living, will pay off.

TALKING AND LISTENING

Conversations at home generally present no problem because usually there are few people and you know who they are. But when you're in a group, even at home, you will need to get people to come over and be close to you if you are to communicate. You cannot call across a room, past others, and hope to be as successful as you might have been as a sighted person.

I found, particularly when I first became blind, that I needed to touch the person to whom I was talking, to assure myself that he or she was facing me and that we were lined up to communicate, so to speak. Many people are reluctant to be touched, I learned, so I became good at asking, "Do you mind if I touch you to get a sense of where you're standing in relation to me? It will help me feel more in contact as we speak." Most people will accept that invitation. To communicate with sighted people it helps if you can come as close as possible to making eye contact, even if you can't see them. If you lift your eyes and look in the direction of the person you are talking to, he or she will feel much more with you.

SEX AND LOVE

How much of the language of love is in the eyes! People communicate their love interest that way. When I was younger and with a young man and we couldn't touch, we would look at each other and be able to see what the other was thinking. But when you're blind you can't communicate that way. Instead of reading facial cues or body language you have to tune into the melody of the voice. What a person says may be interesting, or even loving, but the melody may be cold or abrasive. You learn to listen for warmth, hesitation, interest, all the nuances of feeling that are revealed in the voice and how things are said. When you could see, you still couldn't know for sure. Now you know less. But you can be courageous and guess. It truly is *dancing in the dark.*

Of course there are problems. If you can't see to kiss that special first kiss, it may be aimed wrong. But, practice will make perfect, and that's all I think needs to be said about it! Not everything needs to be expressed tentatively. I know a bold blind man who, taken with me after a lecture I gave, exclaimed: "Come on over here! I want to Braille you!"

There are bound to be some awkward moments. Blind men will reach out, quite innocently, and seem to a sighted woman to be making some kind of advance. Such incidents inevitably happen. They should be handled politely and delicately by both parties, the sighted person suggesting that she doesn't want to be touched at that moment, the blind person apologizing and excusing himself by saying that no offense was intended. In this culture of ours, apparently, sighted women are more often offended in this way by blind men than sighted men by blind women. I wonder why?

I know a professional journalist whose stock-in-trade was reading and writing. As he lost his sight he withdrew more and more from the swirl of the newspaper world that had been his life. He has now withdrawn to such an extent that he's rejected everyone, including people who might serve as readers to him. He knows he's wrong to do this, to be giving up the joy of life to his incapacity. His circle of friends is limited; he surely doesn't date. He's thrown himself away and out of love, because he's out of sight.

I heard about a woman who, after losing her sight, became a hypochondriac to such an extent that she ruined her marriage. When the couple broke up, she dropped the hypochondria. She stopped going to doctors and began to take stock, she went to one little meeting of this group, then another little meeting of that group, and a third little meeting, and so on. She picked up all her old interests: charities, books, and museums. She put the blindness behind her and her best foot forward. She discovered that people paid attention to her. She made new friends, not all blind people either. She went blind into the sighted world and integrated with it. The last I heard, she had broken up with one boyfriend ("too dependent"), and decided that a steady relationship was not for her. She decided to "cut loose."

I'm not endorsing or recommending either alternative, withdrawal or promiscuity. I'm not condemning either. My point is that just as in the sighted world there are all sorts of relationship possibilities, so too in the world of blindness. I have a good friend who's exceedingly kind and generous. We enjoy each other's company. We go to concerts and dinner together, and this involves the usual difficulties: my being sloppy sometimes when eating out and slow in walking down streets. I said to him, "I will ask this only once. I'm so slow, it must be boring and difficult for you. Why do you go out with me?" "I never think about it," he said, "You're just interesting for me to be with and I like you."

Now as to sexual technique, why can't blindness actually improve it? Blindness, in fact, does not get in the way, at least that's what all my many blind friends and acquaintances report. Of course, as you get older, sexual needs are less urgent and people are usually more able to be up front about what they want.

In the end, love is love, the real thing is independent of sightedness or blindness. Helen Keller was blind and had a love life, so did Milton, and Maurice Maeterlinck; why not you and me?

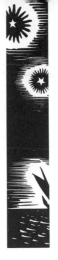

Chapter 5
PUBLIC LIFE:
THE STREET

BECOMING STREETWISE

Because you can't see you are more liable to lose things than sighted people. You may not notice money dropping out of a pocket, for example. Of course you are more vulnerable to thieves. So before you can even think about going out the door you need to make yourself streetwise. The first principle is to distribute your valuables on yourself. The second is to secure them.

Here's how I do it. I have a special inside pocket sewn into all my coats and jackets. In this pocket I keep a small wallet containing my identification and credit cards. For extra safety I prefer to safety pin this little wallet to the pocket.

On the other hand, money that I need to get around with, ready money, I generally keep in two other places. The first is a purse with a strap that I keep on the wrist of the hand in which I hold my cane. The wrist strap acts as one obstacle to my inadvertently letting the purse fall, and the cane acts as a second obstacle. The other place I find useful for "quick money" is a breast pocket. You can't believe how it helps simplify things, giving me access to money without having to open my purse.

Following this rule of distribution of valuables, women can carry keys in yet another place, pinned to your person, not in your jacket which you can easily lose, but pinned, for example, to an inside pocket of your skirt.

Everyone can buy clothing with pockets. Men, of course, have a big advantage here because their clothes tend to come with many more pockets. Men should remember, however, to distribute some of the contents of their wallet to different parts of their person and to avoid using their back pockets. Ready money can go in a shirt or jacket pocket. Change can go in another jacket pocket, and so on.

WALKING ON THE STREET

A white cane comes in handy because it helps you find obstacles in your path. A white cane also signals to passersby that you are blind and may need help. Don't be afraid to speak up. Asking for help is a reality. Generally, people are willing to help you.

When you ask, be explicit: "Excuse me, I am blind." Avoid understatement, unnecessary tact, or anything resembling circumlocution. Even saying "I cannot see" may not get the point across. "I am blind" will do nicely. In short: don't deny yourself to get yourself around.

Sometimes you'll have to repeat yourself, when you ask directions, for instance. You might say, "Is such-and-such street to my left or right?" The hurrying sighted person might have an impulse to point or nod and simply add, "It's over there." Just as you have a right to say you're blind and to be explicit, you have a right to repeat yourself: "I'm sorry, sir, I'm blind. Is it to my left or right?"

As a general rule you need to trust these strangers on the street. You can't do much else, really. Sometimes they will offer to accompany you, and that is very nice indeed. You'd be surprised how kind people are.

Of course not everyone is solicitous of the blind. I've had to learn how to deal with panhandlers, sometimes unscrupulous ones. Blind people just cannot allow themselves to respond to an unknown solicitation for money in the street. You are too vulnerable. So you must never reveal where you keep your valuables. One Sunday morning, when my friend Jim and I were walking down the street, Jim, who can still see very dimly, made out someone approaching and could tell that it was a well dressed person. The fellow stopped us and asked for money. Can you imagine! He was a wise guy to boot. "Can you help me?" he whined. "I put my last penny in the collection plate!" Obviously, on a Sunday, with a church nearby, and we being two older and conservatively dressed people, he thought a churchy appeal would be just the thing. But I had been tipped off by Jim to the fellow's clothes. So I just raised my cane and shouted: "Can't you see we're blind!" He retreated from us as if my cane were a snake! I don't usually handle beggars this harshly, but, I repeat, you've got to be careful and not enter into a relationship with them.

Sometimes, when walking with a friend, my vanity takes over. I fold up my cane so that people won't notice I am blind. After all, I want to look just like everybody else. For example, when my friend Joe takes me to dinner, I don't want to look blind, I'm on a big date! But pride can go before a fall. If you do this sort of thing, be as careful as I am. I tell Joe, for instance, "I'm putting my cane away and I'm relying on you. Tell me when there's a step up, step down, or any kind of obstruction. Otherwise, I'll just walk half a step behind you and I'll follow you and do what you do." I also ask my friend to precede me through a doorway, opening the door but not holding it open. I hold it open with one hand, and with the other I reach for my companion, then we'll walk together again. For this reason, obviously, I ask gentlemen friends not to be polite, because if they held the door open for me I'd be going along by myself once past the door, and that could be scary.

If you have friends who will walk with you, you can get a chance to play. For instance, I like to walk quickly; it's fun for me. I have a friend who takes me to a promenade in my city. Once there I put my cane away, take his hand, and walk boldly and freely for as many as five blocks because there are no curbs and no steps. This is truly a great pleasure for me. To top it off, we'll sit on a bench at the end of the walkway and I'll just listen to the sounds of the sea, the birds, the boats, and smell the ocean. I don't often get a chance to walk so freely, and so I cherish these opportunities.

I have another sighted guide, my friend Ethan, who is five years old. He loves my cane. He loves to collapse and extend it. He has great fun telling me what's ahead, and even greater fun leading me. He walks ahead of me with the cane extended before him and I follow with my hand on his head. So wherever he goes, I go. I trust him and we both get a great sense of accomplishment from our walks this way. My granddaughter, being very close to me, is more playful with me than most other people dare to be. In some ways she pushes my limits, and that can be great fun. When we're walking, she likes to start running. Well, so do I. Because I trust her, I can fly. A storekeeper said to me after one of these flights (I was over seventy years old at the time), "Why were you running?" I said, "I wasn't running, she was. I just followed." Then we all laughed. Sometimes she even teases me, "Stop! A hole!" she says, and she laughs and confesses after I screech to a halt, "I was just teasing." We laughed again.

Of course, there are many times when one doesn't want to walk or just can't take the trouble. In my city, San Francisco, cabs are a marvelous convenience for the blind, though they can be costly. When I'm tired or fed up or the weather turns bad my cane becomes my precious ally. It signals the cabby to come out and help me, and of course I tend to get preferential treatment when there is competition for cabs, for example on rainy days.

The driver will usually get out at the end of the ride and escort me to the curb or even to my door. At which point I might take his shoulder or his hand and say, "See, there are some good things about being blind. Just look at this, I'm getting to hold hands with a strange fellow, and that's nice." I'll pause for a moment and then really lay it on thick, because I so much enjoy the special freedom that blindness gives me to flirt. "You know, even though I can't see you, I know that you're young and handsome." Actually, I say this to many men, and they love it. Some say, "Yes, I'm young, but not handsome." Others say, "Yes, I'm handsome, but not young." The best of all is when one says, "How did you guess?" and some, naturally, say, "No, no. Now I really know you're blind!" It's great fun, and I really wouldn't carry on this way if I weren't blind.

The advantages of blindness: *never underestimate the possibilities for flirting.*

CROSSING THE STREET

You've exited your house and made it to the corner. But now you must cross the street. The crowd is moving across. Do you move with them? No. You wait. Listen for the stop of oncoming traffic, and as you cross you hold your cane slightly lifted and moving. Moving your cane attracts the attention of the people you want to see you: oncoming pedestrians and drivers. Don't, however, hold the cane straight out in front, you can skewer people that way, and such acts are very bad publicity for the blind!

Some people at an intersection wave their canes overhead, like a flag. One of my acquaintances does that when she crosses Market Street in San Francisco, a six-lane affair with two sets of trolley car tracks as well as separate lanes for buses. Don't hesitate to call attention to yourself in such situations.

Speaking of canes and meeting the public, you must be prepared for surprises and accept them. I know a blind executive

45

who was extremely successful in his work and had a top management post in a major government department in Washington D.C. He knew the intersections between his office and home very well and was used to navigating them easily in practically all weather. One sunny day he felt the end of his cane being lifted in front of him and himself being forced to follow across the street, "half-led, half-dragged," as he complained to me, "like a donkey!" He was infuriated at the indignity but, he told me afterward, "I just said thank you and let the fellow go about his business." His point was that even though some people may not use their own eyes to see you clearly and know that you are a thinking person and an individual, it's good not to be too thin-skinned. It's important that the blind maintain good public relations, and besides, it's courteous to acknowledge a well-intentioned gesture even if it was momentarily irritating.

I had a teacher who taught me the basics of walking on the street. He taught me to measure the distance down from the curb with my cane. Something as complicated as learning to walk on your own on the street takes a lot of courage and practice, by yourself or with a friend. The most basic and important thing, however, is to just get yourself out there, you'll find the information you need to put it together in your own way.

GETTING ON THE BUS

After you have found the bus stop, you've got to make sure you get on the right bus. You can't see the number so you ask someone standing in line, or the driver, "Is this the number 43?" More often than not you will simply get a nod or a shake of the head for an answer. Rephrase the question so that it will necessarily get an answer you can grasp, a verbal one: "What bus number is this?" If your condition is not perfectly obvious, be explicit: "I'm blind, can you tell me what bus this is, please?"

Once you know you're getting on the right bus, tell the driver, "I am blind. I cannot see. Can you please signal me when we're at the corner of Fifth and Mission Streets?" Notice how this is different from "Will you tell me when we're at the corner of Fifth and Mission because I can't read the sign." It may be clear to you what "I can't read the sign" means, but it may not be strong enough to get through to a busy bus driver who has to keep his eyes off his passengers and on the road. So feel free to be direct and emphatic. Rephrase your request along the lines I'm suggesting, "Driver, I'm blind. I can't see. . ." Let people know you'll be in trouble unless they help out.

GETTING OFF THE BUS

I remember once, as a passenger, I had asked to be signaled for my stop, but the bus driver forgot. I ended up being left off seven blocks too far, obviously a significant additional problem if one is blind. You have a right to remind the driver where you want to get off. The trick is to remind, but politely. And, as always, to get people's attention it helps to give them a name or a title: "Driver, are we approaching such-and-such street?" Or, "Sir," addressing another passenger if the bus driver is busy, "will you please tell me where we are now?"

THE SUBWAY

In general it is people who have been blind from birth and had extensive hands-on training from an early age who use the subways. People blinded later in life, especially senior citizens, have a hard time making the adjustments and learning the skills needed. That doesn't mean one can't try, but this is an area in which special and careful instruction is required. The following anecdote illustrates this.

I know a man who wanted the experience of using the subway. He was at his doctor's office. The doctor said, "I'm closing the office soon. Why don't you wait and I'll take you?" So after the last patient left, the doctor accompanied him down to the station and got him into the subway car. "You go to the next to the last stop on the line," he said, and then simply left. I'll never forget my friend's words: "Finding a seat was easy. But I had no idea when I would get to the next-to-the-last stop, so I had to ask. When I hurried off, lest the doors close on me, I was half-frantic, I had to round people up. 'Where am I; Where's the staircase?' When I finally got to the street I had to stop people and begin to navigate all over again. 'Now where am I?' It was a wild experience. Very difficult. But I did it. I guess I did it, by guess, and the seat of my pants, by golly."

This man chuckles at the recollection now, but there are some important lessons for us in the incident. One, we must explain to sighted people exactly what we need in the way of directions. But an equally important lesson is that it takes courage to learn new things. It's true the man said it was a "wild experience" and that he would never do it again. But he did do it and he was proud. He knows and reaffirms that for a blind person it simply takes extra effort to do anything.

STAIRS AND HANDRAILS, ESCALATORS AND ELEVATORS

Steps need not be a problem. The first thing to realize, however, is that sighted people and blind people may often count steps differently. I'm walking downstairs with a friend. She says, "There are four steps down." I've learned to pay little attention to such statements. I rely on my cane and the railing. Sighted people most often will count treads, not risers. But four treads down may really mean five risers (five steps). I ask people to tell me when I'm on the top level.

Between a skillfully used cane and a handrail, a blind person can negotiate steps rather easily. Handrails tell stories. They tell where the stairs begin and end, but not always. Sometimes architects start their handrails two steps after the beginning and end them two steps before the end. In certain public buildings, the San Francisco Opera House is one, you might break your neck if you try relying on handrails alone.

Approach escalators with caution and with the help of a friend. Keep your cane away from the moving steps. Tell your friend, in advance, that you want her to put your hand lightly on the handrail and at an appropriate moment to say, "And step!" At that moment, you step on. When the moment is approaching to get off she should give you some advance notice, and again, at the right time, you move when she says, "And step off!"

I try to use elevators when there are people around me so that I know the right button is pushed and there's someone to tell me when to get off. However, there are elevators today which electronically beep to indicate the passing of floors.

Chapter 6
PUBLIC LIFE: SHOPPING

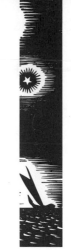

Now that you are able to navigate in the public world, you can use your newly and gradually acquired abilities to take care of your needs and pleasures. For that, you must relate to the world as a new kind of consumer, a blind shopper.

Essential shopping when you are blind is mainly of two kinds: marketing for food and household supplies, and buying clothing and other things that you are liable to find in big stores, especially department stores.

MARKETING FOR FOOD AND HOUSEHOLD SUPPLIES

People who still have some vision left can usually navigate pretty well by themselves in supermarkets. If they can still read the names on bottles and cans, they can take a monocular to the store. This is a cross between a jeweler's loupe and a telescope, one to three inches long, which you use to read things in the middle distance, for instance, something on a shelf two feet up. You hold the monocular to your eye, and if your vision is strong enough it will allow you to tell a can of chicken soup from pea soup. For close observation, where you can really get near what you are trying to read or identify, you can use a magnifying glass. These come in all sorts of sizes, shapes and strengths, and some are equipped with a built-in flashlight to further increase visibility.

People who can use this sort of equipment are probably best off doing their marketing in one or two stores that they know well. It's hell to market in places you don't know. Of course, even in these familiar places, you need to learn the aisles and the placement of types of food. A good part of the time, for example, you can tell an item by size and shape and can distinguish a quart of milk from a half-gallon. But you may not be able to tell a quart of milk from a quart of Half-and-Half, or packaged butter from margarine. If you know the place where you shop well and if you can still see a little bit and have your magnifiers and monocular, you can, after practicing, actually shop by yourself.

I've got a friend with a three-and-a-half-inch telescope. There she stands in an aisle looking through it, saying to herself, "I look like a captain gazing out to sea!" But one day the shop owner came up to her and asked what she was doing. He seemed suspicious, even irate. She told him and he said, "Oh, I'm sorry, I thought you were a shoplifter!"

A Philosophy For Shopping, as Well as For Life

The above story illustrates what is perhaps the basic rule for all kinds of shopping: make yourself known. Just like on the street or in the bus, you need to explain yourself whenever you walk into a store. "I'm a low vision person. I'll need help. Can you help me find things?" Or, "if I bring them to you, can you help me sort them out to be sure they're exactly what I want?" As we go along, I'll continue to stress how important it is to speak up in this way.

Now, and this is also a constant refrain in this book, everyone will have to find his or her own way. I make suggestions, sometimes very detailed ones, the rest is up to you. You do the best you can with the sight you have. What I give you here are not rules, not exact guidelines. You have to do some work on your own, to improvise, and also to ask for help. A good practice, while you read this book, is to put it down after every page or section or chapter and ask yourself, "How does this fit in with my life? Can I think of other ideas, better ones than Frances', to get better results in the same area?" One reason this book is so detailed about living blind is to show you how to do it. Another reason, equally important, is to get you to think about how to do it better. My whole philosophy is that life is creative and that living with blindness gives us a wonderful opportunity to be inventive. We can become the engineers and artists of a new kind of life.

The advantages of blindness: *it gives us a wonderful opportunity to be inventive.*

Shopping List
Here are my six steps for food shopping:

Step 1: I make a shopping list on my tape recorder. Once I've got all the items on tape, I play it back and write them down. For me this takes time, sometimes a lot. I write them down on a piece of paper. If there's a friend around to do this for me of course it's going to be more legible, because sometimes what I write is just indecipherable.

Step 2: I call the supermarket. I say something like "I'm blind, and I need some help when I come in to shop. Do you have someone to give me this special customer service and assist me?"

Most big stores have customers' helpers, but many people don't realize that such services are available and that one can get fabulous assistance if you ask for it. If the answer is "Yes, we can help you," then I ask, "What time are you least busy? What time would be most convenient?" I'm trying to accommodate myself to the reality of the situation, to arrive when there are the fewest customers so I can get the most attention from the personnel. In other words, I want to go when someone can really give me time and won't be too hurried and won't, in turn, be hurrying me. I know a blind woman who went to a store at a peak time with a long list. The manager would not help her. "We're too busy now." So she needed to make a whole new trip because she failed to call first. For the blind, it's good advice to continually plan ahead."

Step 3: I enter, find my way to the checkout counter, and say, "I'm blind. I'm here with my list. I called earlier. Is there anyone here who can help me?"

Step 4: Here comes the person who will either take my list or go around with me. Personally, I mostly prefer not to go around the store. "Let them pick it out" is my philosophy. But others may well feel differently.

Step 5: Before the helper goes off, I ask that person to read me the list. That way, we are both clear about exactly what's on it.

Step 6: The helper comes back bringing the food and other supplies. "Let's check," I say. "Let's read the list and go through the items in the basket." Sometimes the customers' helper will have forgotten something, or sometimes I'll have forgotten to list a particular item. Sometimes the helper will describe a size or a brand and it won't be what I want: a pint for a quart or a brand of ketchup that I hate. Once I wanted applesauce but neglected to say I wanted it strained, and the person brought chunky. It was my fault. Once I wanted a dehydrated soup of a certain brand. He got those points right, but brought tomato instead of split pea. Another time when the helper brought thin spaghetti instead of medium, I had compassion and decided it didn't matter so much. It's my right to get the merchandise I want, I know, but I'm also aware that I must not be too picky, the next time the whole staff might be reluctant to help.

So marketing is a slow process that can be painstaking and sometimes even difficult. It requires patience. But mostly it will be pleasant, and very important, it allows you to keep your independence.

Let *patience, organization, and independence* be one of your refrains.

THE MEAT COUNTER

The meat and poultry counter is a special matter. You need to make a separate call ahead before you go to the store. You say, "I'm the blind lady who was in last month, do you remember me? By the way, what's your name? Bob? Well hello, Bob. Do you have time to talk to me now?" If Bob says "Yes," I'm ready. I have made my list in advance and there is no hesitation. "Bob, can you prepare the following items for me?" He may say that if I come in at such-and-such a time he can wait on me and tell me all the specials. If he does, I express my pleasure and look him up when I'm at the store.

This can, however, get complicated, calling for your usual flexibility. Once when I came and Bob wasn't there, the butcher who waited on me said, "Lady, I don't have time for this." I got firm: "If you don't, find me a butcher who does."

Well, he did. But there is the same old lesson here. Though I was right to be firm, I made the mistake of not identifying myself as a low vision person. He thought I was sighted and asking for unnecessary extra help. By the time I told him I couldn't see, he had already dismissed me as a sighted person who wanted too much service.

So the meat counter is a good place to remind ourselves of the importance of good communication skills and, in particular, the need to be precise and explicit. Once I told my butcher that I wanted "two pieces of very tender steak, each piece to weigh no more than three-quarters of a pound. It's no use you showing it to me, I can't see, I am blind." "Fine," said the butcher, "How do you want them cut?" "Cut them each in half," I replied. "Do you want the halves cut?" he asked. I didn't think twice about saying, "No, thank you. Once is enough." But when I got home, I discovered the pieces were very thick.

Obviously, I should have picked up on his question and asked him why he was asking me about cutting the halves in half. But I didn't. I think there are two important lessons here. First, you can't always think of everything. So be prepared to forgive yourself. Second, you have the right to ask a second question. You have the right to ask as many questions as you need. Speak up. Take your time. Don't be afraid. Too often both sighted and blind people are afraid to ask questions. I keep telling myself that it is okay not to know and okay to ask. After all, we are all floating in the same murky sea and doing the best crawl stroke we can. So be pleasant–but ask! This is one of the advantages of blindness: *you aren't expected to know everything, so you can give yourself permission to ask more readily than sighted people.*

CHECKOUT

The next step, of course, is getting through the checkout counter. Have the clerks pack all your groceries in your shopping cart. Finally, you must pay, but how? By check? Very difficult. Do you sign it after someone else fills it out? Well, that can be dangerous. You also have the problem of entering the amount of the check in your checkbook and calculating your new balance. Cash is good. So are credit cards. My own favorite is to use traveler's checks. It's the next best thing to cash, but you don't have to worry about losing them or keeping your bank balance. Then you get cash back by way of change. I always have twenty- or fifty-dollar traveler's checks in my purse. If my purchases come to $38.50, I don't have to struggle with filling out a check. I sign my name and get change.

GETTING HOME

At last you are ready to leave the store. Do you call a cab? You can ask the manager to make the call for you. Or you may have made an appointment with a driver or a friend to pick you up. Can you get home on your own? Do you call a volunteer service? These exist in some cities and you can find them through community, church, or social service organizations.

There's no one to parent you. You do the best you can with what you've got.

SHOPPING IN OTHER KINDS OF STORES

Whether you're shopping for clothing or cutlery, you'll need special help. Most department stores have customized shopping services. Call ahead for an appointment. Most of the time, if you have explained yourself clearly by saying you are "blind and cannot see," you can give the person sizes, colors, and styles of the items you want over the phone. When you get there the customers' helper will show you a variety of things from which you can choose. I once went into a store to buy a coffee maker. I must have asked maybe a hundred and twenty questions until I settled on a make and style of machine that would be easy for me to operate. That's the way to do it. Ask plenty of questions until you find out exactly what you need and which item will be satisfactory.

Shopping By Phone

Often you can do specialty shopping by phone without even going to the store. The whole institution of 800 numbers is a godsend for the blind. Before you order an item, have these things in mind: the brand you want, the style, the size, the color, and every other pertinent detail. Many telephone customer service people are rather good at helping you get to this point. With others, you may need more persistence and patience. If you're not succeeding feel free to ask to talk with a supervisor or another representative. Ultimately, however, it is your responsibility to clearly say what you want. You must know what you are looking for and understand the range of available options. So, get your act together as much as you can before you call.

Again, it goes back to what I've said before: *Organization, Organization, Organization!*

Advantages of Small Shops

If you are particular about how you look, as most of us are, you may find it most effective to buy your clothing from smaller stores. Here you can get to know the owner or one or two clerks who, in turn, can get to know you. Over time they will learn your tastes and be able to help you find what you want quickly. As with bus and taxicab drivers, make a point of being friendly. Once you have made this sort of connection you can call up and say, "I want to buy a wool skirt and a cotton blouse, of such-and-such a color, for such-and-such an occasion. Do you have anything that you think will work for me?" If they say they do, you arrange to come in, as with the supermarket, when they are not busy so they can give you the special attention you require. Once I get there I don't automatically accept the first thing they offer. But I do, in some measure, have to rely on them. I can specify price and function, I can feel whether the texture is one I like, I can determine the size I need. But, unless I bring a friend with me, I have to rely on the salespeople for style and color. Because I do rely on them I need to know them. When I enter a store for the first time, understanding as I do that I need clerks to know and help me over the long haul, I approach the whole enterprise as an adventure in making friends. I make sure to ask their names, I tell them mine, I explain that I'm blind, I take the opportunity to chat with them, and then I ask them if they have what I want.

For example, they may offer me a selection of skirts. I choose the one I want and ask the clerk to find a blouse that goes with it. And slowly and calmly, we'll go through the whole selection process together, the salesperson taking the time to do for me that which I cannot do for myself. I have come out with some pretty outfits this way, or so I have been told by friends. People often ask me how I manage to buy things that are color-coordinated. When I get the outfit home, I take a single hanger so my gorgeous ensemble will all be in one place. I make sure to get all the tags off right away—to forget is to end up wearing your best outfit with those things flapping around you.

The advantages of blindness: *you get waited on and get help with things you used to have to do by yourself.*

DELIVERIES

Personally, I no longer have my groceries delivered. I found that when the delivery person left I had a pile of objects and not the vaguest idea of what was what. In addition, I did not like having a delivery person fill out my check.

When it comes to simple purchases, from the druggist, for example, I rely on deliveries. I call and ask how much the bill will be and then have the exact amount ready for the delivery person and, always, some kind of tip.

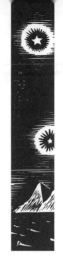

Chapter 7
Public Life: the Bank, the Post Office, and Public Restrooms

Banking and Cash

In banks, as in stores, it's personal contact that will get things done for you. Over the years of trying to deal with banking as a low vision person, I have found it's best not to bother with waiting in line for a teller. Instead, I get to know the manager or the assistant manager by name, and I make my deposits or withdrawals or any other transactions at that person's desk. These people are willing to help and not only do I ask them to take care of the particular transaction, I also bring my deposit books, my check register, and any other documents I need assistance with. I tell them: "Not only are you my bankers, you're also my bookies!" After all, I explain, they keep my accounts straight for me.

By now it shouldn't surprise anyone when I say that it's my practice, as with other service people, to call my banker ahead of time and ask when would be convenient for my visit. When I call, I let her know the information and help I will need so that I can be in and out quickly and don't use too much of her time.

One thing I have learned is to avoid banks around the first of the month, everyone is terribly busy at that time with incoming government checks and other monthly matters. Also, I've found it convenient to have the checks due me made payable to the bank for my account. That way I don't have to deal with a lot of checks coming through my hands. Another tip: Your bank can provide you with a number of ways of facilitating writing checks. They can give you a "check-writing guide," so that you can write in between the lines. I don't like to have a top line to contain my writing so I don't order these. They can also give you printed checks with raised lines. I have other people fill out my checks, but I have them printed with the signature line raised so that I can sign my name easily.

When I go into the bank simply for cash I'm always very careful. Personally, I prefer only to deal with one and five dollar bills. I tell the manager or assistant manager at the desk how much cash I want, say, a hundred dollars. I will make clear that I want the hundred dollars in five-dollar bills. Then when he is counting out the money, I ask him to stop after he gets to twenty-five dollars. I fold them in a way I like, put a clip on them, and then I know I have twenty-five dollars. Then he'll count out a second set of five-dollar bills, and I'll fold and clip them too and so have a second set of twenty-five dollars. And so on, until I have my four little sets of twenty-five dollars each. I find these relatively easy to handle for cash transactions.

Each person will have his or her own system of handling money. My system is to have a snap purse with three compartments in it. One compartment holds a clip of twenty-five dollars. In the middle compartment I keep only dollar bills, which I fold in a different way from five-dollar bills. And in the third section I have five-dollar bills but not in bundles of twenty-five. From here I can quickly pull a five out if I need to without having to take it off the clip. So I have a very good sense of how many fives and ones I have besides my clip of twenty-five dollars. If this sort of thing works for you, fine. If not, do it your own way. One woman I know uses several sets of very thin wallets: one for ones, one for fives, and so forth.

As for coins, I have found that to be a long-term project. By now I have learned that quarters and dimes have milled edges, nickels and pennies have smooth edges. I have also learned that a nickel is a little bit larger than a penny and also a little bit thicker. Most of the time when I need to give anyone change, I simply pour whatever there is in my change purse into my hand and say, "Help yourself." I rarely take the time to identify coins because it's time-consuming and I would rather spend my time identifying paper money.

Here again, this is just my way of doing things. Once I gave a blind friend of mine a dollar folded my particular way. He said, "You're giving me a twenty, not a one." "In my world," I answered, "that is the way I fold ones." "Oh," he replied, "according to my own private way of doing things, that's a twenty." So you see, everyone works out these details of living in his or her own way.

What is useful here for you? What do you want to remember? What other ways of doing these things can you think of?

POST OFFICE

This is at once a small and a large subject. In the first place, every blind person is entitled to a rubber stamp with the words "Free Matter for the Blind." This can be used to send large print, taped, or Braille material. If somebody is writing a letter for you, you may, if you sign it, also use the stamp. Of course, I always keep a roll of stamps on hand because I often mail things that have nothing to do with my disability and then the rubber stamp may not be used. Check these regulations with your post office.

On occasion, when I am expecting a package but will not be home, I'll call the post office, explain that I am blind, and ask them to have the carrier leave the package outside my door. I explain that going to the post office is a burden and that I will take responsibility for any loss. Sometimes a carrier will get to know me and if I'm not home he will leave the package by the door automatically, because we have an understanding.

Unless your mail is in Braille, you need someone to read it for you. The fact that you have to have your mail read diminishes your privacy. Your personal mail, your junk mail, your bills, all of it is no longer your own. The only way you can have real privacy in correspondence is to receive your letters on tape so you can listen in your own solitary corner to whatever it is your friend has to say. And, by the same token, you can communicate with that person through tapes of your own.

Because correspondence is so cumbersome, the blind person has to rely on the phone even more than most people do. The phone company facilitates this, in part, by allowing you to use Information and Operator Assistance without charge. Do make sure you take advantage of this service. Call your telephone billing office and have the fact that you are blind registered on your billing information. Then, whenever you call information or need operator assistance, just tell the operator you are blind or "this is a manual call," and you will not be charged.

PUBLIC RESTROOMS

This is, in all polite company, a delicate topic. But blind people must be brave!

You might need a public restroom almost anywhere: in the waiting room of a railroad terminal or airport, in a restaurant, at a theater or museum, and so on. What to do? You ask someone to help and get yourself escorted to it. Generally, a service person connected with the facility, a flight attendant or porter, for example, will be available to do this for you.

Once you have been taken to the door, unless you're sure of the layout inside, it's best to wait until you hear someone else entering and ask, "Excuse me, will you please help me into the restroom?" After you go in, you can also ask to be shown to a stall. This is a situation where people are particularly inclined to be helpful. They understand the obvious real need and, as long as you're gentle in your request, they will help you.

I usually ask where the flush handle is. Some are in odd places, like in the wall above or below the seat. In planes or trains especially, this can be a problem.

Sinks can also be a problem. Some blind people skip washing up because it's a lot to deal with, different types of faucets (one for hot and cold together or one for each, the kind you press, the kind you turn, the kind you lift), different types of soap dispensers, paper towel dispensers, those electric fan dryers, and so on. If someone else is around, don't be ashamed to ask for help. Asking for help is your standard resource.

Sometimes public facilities can be an amusing area for visually impaired people. One young woman waiting in an airport lounge had just enough vision to recognize a famous senator, a man she thought of as a great benefactor to his constituency. He turned away and began walking rapidly, just after she spied him. Excited at the chance to meet him the woman went in pursuit. He entered a room; she followed. He turned abruptly toward her. She extended her right hand and declared, "Senator, you've done so much for so many, I want to shake your hand." "Wait for me outside, young woman," he replied rather firmly, "this is the men's room!" Imagine her confusion, consternation, and embarrassment! Well, she got over them fast and, with almost instant presence of mind, accepted the humor of the event, explained she didn't see very well, and made her way out as gracefully as she could. They both laughed about it a few minutes afterward and she got an autograph as a souvenir.

As a blind person you have to be prepared to accept such occasional blunders in a good spirit. A man who has been blind most of his life confided to me that he has sometimes mistaken a sink for a urinal, only figuring out the mistake when he reached forward for the flush and discovered a faucet.

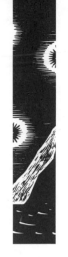

Chapter 8
SOCIALIZING

Socializing means entertaining at home. It also means going out to parties and restaurants and public entertainments, meetings, and generally being with people. This is fun time.

AT HOME

Socializing at home is easy. I can pick my spot and invite a friend to sit wherever she or he wants to, and so we can talk easily. If we need a snack or a drink, I say to my friend, "Well, what will you have? There's tea or coffee and cookies. Please help yourself from that cabinet and help me too." It works out very well. People are very willing to help themselves. You don't have to serve people in order to be a good host and for them to have a good time at your home. Be honest about what you need and all will go smoothly. You can even invite people to take a look in your cupboards and see what they might want. Do this, because for a blind person out of sight is often out of mind. No one can remember everything on the shelves but you can remember to tell your friend where the cupboards are and where various kinds of items are located. From then on, it's very easy.

It is possible to go beyond having just a few people over, blind people can have parties. Of course, you can't do this entirely on your own. Recently I enlisted a couple of people to help and gave a pancake party. First, being a good organizer, I got straight what I wanted to serve in the way of food, how I wanted it laid out, whom I wanted to invite. Then I asked a friend who helps in the house to come put out the dishes and do the cooking. My granddaughter Christine helped too. She was a great flipper of pancakes that morning. The menu was pancakes and sausage, mimosa cocktails, fruit salad and yogurt, coffee and tea. Forty people arrived over a period of hours that Sunday.

It was great fun, of course, but I want to make two points. First, part of the success of the party came from mixing up the sighted and the non-sighted people. In order to get there, most blind people had to have a sighted friend accompany them. This works to the advantage of both. The sighted person feels a kind of pleasant obligation toward the unsighted friend and new companions, and the unsighted people have a sense of comfort that they're not alone, lost and unseeing, in a swirling crowd of sound and bodies. The second point has to do with one of my pet themes—flirting. As a blind person I never miss a chance at any social occasion, my own parties particularly, to take advantage of the special variety of flirting that blindness allows. One of the blind men was leaving and he called out to me, "Good-bye, Frances. Nice party, see you again." I was sitting with a group of women, as it happened, but I hastened to say to them, "Oh, excuse me for a moment. I've got to feel George good-bye." I thought that was a very funny line. There's a hint there for everyone. Well, if you're a man, you have to be more reticent about feeling the girls good-bye. That is, I take advantage of my blindness to do a lot of wholesome hugging, any blind person can do the same. In fact, everyone, blind or not, might consider doing it.

GOING OUT

It's a little harder going to someone else's house. In your own house all the guests are invited by you. You know who's there and they all come to you, wherever you are, because you're the host. But, being blind in another person's house, you can't simply walk up to someone spontaneously and say, "Hi, I haven't seen you for a long time." Nor can you nudge a companion and whisper, "Who's that person over there?" You can't initiate social contact in this way, you need to wait for people to come to you.

If you're with a friend you can say, "Listen, sit me down, or bring me over to so-and-so. Then you can take off. Just keep an eye on me and make sure I don't get stuck by myself doing nothing. Check in on me in, say, five minutes or so." Your friend and you know very well that you cannot walk around the room. You are a stuck person.

When I first lost most of my vision I didn't have the courage to negotiate social gatherings. After all, I didn't necessarily know the people, I couldn't see, and I couldn't circulate. But I learned to make the most of just sitting. For instance, I practiced starting up conversations.

If you sense somebody next to you, you might say "Hi, I'm Frances. As my white cane tells you, I can't see you. What's your name?" Sometimes you'll discover that you're talking to somebody's back or, horror of horrors, interrupting a conversation. If that happens, just apologize and go on from there, whether they are turned toward you or away from you. Just going on is the name of the socializing game.

Sometimes if you start a conversation in this way you may even find, it has often happened to me, that you're the center of a small group of people who are happy to have someone draw them into conversation instead of themselves having the hard job of striking up conversations with strangers. If you're going to become a professional icebreaker like this, and there is every reason to do so, you learn the basic gambits: "Hi, what's your name?" "What brings you here?" So begins a whole conversation. Sighted people use the same maneuvers, but you have the disadvantage of not being able to see if the person you're talking with is interested or looks as if they would rather be somewhere else. As always, be absolutely honest and realistic and say, at an appropriate moment, "If you have to go off at any point, please feel free, but just tell me you are going."

When I meet people, or for that matter when I'm saying good-bye, I always extend my hand first. Thus I avoid the embarrassment of not finding the person's hand. This is another example of how I have had to learn to be socially more forward than I might have been when sighted. I count it on the plus side of being blind. Making physical contact in this way is another plus. It compensates, in part, for not being able to see. You can learn a lot about people just by paying attention to hands, their energy, temperature, texture, and so on. Being blind pushes you to overcome shyness and to be a "social activist."

Whether it is a large swirling cocktail party or a smaller gathering I find I manage well if I go with one or two people. Once I get myself located I relieve my original escorts of their burden and I do my best on my own. If somebody hands me a drink and I've got it but don't know where to put it, I just ask, "Will someone please put this drink down for me?" Sometimes I talk too much or too loud and don't realize it. Sometimes I'm a pain. But sometimes I'm a pleasure! The only way I've figured out to stay afloat in social life is to say to myself, as I say to you: "Try to swim, even if you can only do the dog paddle."

Now your socializing is not always done in the sighted or mixed world. There is the social world of the blind, too. Here things can be a little different, often delightfully so. For instance, I was invited to address a meeting of people who had recently lost their sight and were having a difficult time read-justing and reintegrating into the sighted world. One of the men said to me, "How can you tell the age of a person to whom you're speaking?" "To tell you the truth," I replied, "I never thought of that. I listen to what the person is saying and respond according-ly and never think about how old the person is. By the way, as long as we're on the subject, and I won't be hurt by your answer, how old do you think I am?" Now this man was as blind as I was, but he was still in the guessing stage of finding his way through life. "Well," said he, "I take you to be fifty-five." "You're off by twenty years," I said. "Are you seventy-five?" he asked, which is the case. "What's the matter with you?" I exclaimed. "Can't you subtract?" Among blind people, this sort of thing is a good enough joke. We both had quite a nice laugh at that one.

ENTERTAINMENT: THE PERFORMING ARTS

The most important thing about going to any sort of performance is to find out as much as you can in advance. It helps to be familiar with the setting, the libretto, etc., so that your mind has something to relate to from the moment you walk in. Even if you go to a play that you don't know too much about, a new drama, for instance, if you listen closely you'll get a pretty good idea of what's going on. Comedies can be less satisfying to a blind person because seeing the nonverbal cues is often essential to getting what's funny. On the other hand, theatrical events involving monologue or dialogue are very easy to follow. So is stand-up comedy, except for the sight gags. In any case, sit back and let whatever it is flow over you. What you don't understand, what you miss, you can ask a friend about at intermission. Or you can just forget it and take what you can. You'll get much more than you could imagine in this relaxed way.

Musical performances, thank goodness, are for the ear. So you're ahead of the game there if you know what the composition is and can recognize the instruments. For me a ballet is out of the question. I never liked it even when I could see, so I just listen to the music and let it go at that.

In general, for all performing arts events, I go with the flow. I prepare myself as best I can, I try not to get frustrated at what I might miss, and above all, I let myself enjoy whatever comes through for me. That's the secret.

You can even go to baseball games. You miss a lot of it, of course, but at least you have the fun of being out there, part of the crowd. If the game is being broadcast, you can follow it on a little transistor radio.

I've gone to dances, blind as I am, both with a sighted companion and a low vision companion. I have quite a good time if I trust my companion, that's essential. I listen closely to the beat and everything works out fine. Truly *dancing in the dark.*

THE MUSEUM

Among my greatest sorrows is not being able to see the beauty of color and composition in art. Even the loss of reading is nothing compared to this, because I have taught myself Braille and I have audio cassettes. It's just darn hard to find a companion who will take you to a museum and patiently describe things to you, and it's just as hard, if not more so, to find one who has a talent for it. It isn't quite as difficult, however, with sculpture. The most comfortable place for me is a hands-on show.

Going to an art exhibition with another low vision person has its special comforts, such as pacing ourselves to our own abilities. Whether you are with a sighted or unsighted companion, you can ask so much more and the experience can be very rich. Whole aspects of life go on around us and pass us by because we don't ask or don't know what to ask. *Ask, Ask, Ask!* Within reason, of course. You need to be concerned about intruding on the privacy and time and personal enjoyment of a sighted person, but I have sighted friends who positively delight in going to the museum with me because it helps them to see. Obviously, the effort to articulate what one sees to someone who can't see sharpens perception, analysis, and appreciation.

RESTAURANTS AND DINING OUT

It used to be that when I was first blind I would only order scallops as a main course: they were easy to spear with a fork. I also used to always order soup as a first course because it was easy to spoon up. I used to skip bread and butter because buttering the bread was a production. I never ordered any kind of meat because I couldn't easily use a knife and fork and I never used to order chicken because of the bones I would have to fight with.

But those days are all over now. I know what to do, and I know how to ask specifically for what I need. If I order chicken I ask the chef or the waiter to cut it into bite-size pieces. The same with steak or other kinds of meat. I emphasize "bite-size pieces" to them, having already identified myself as a low vision person and explained why I am asking for this special help. In fact, if there is anything that I order which I can't handle by finger or by fork, I have it cut for me. I'll even ask for a salad to be cut up. Sometimes, if I get the sense that they'll enjoy the joke, I tell people, "I'm not the old cut-up I used to be," anything to get a laugh and make it easier for people to feel relaxed and enjoy helping out, and to help me feel relaxed.

I have gotten less squeamish about using my fingers to help me eat in public. I explain to my companions: "You'll notice I'm using my fingers to eat. But fingers were invented before forks!" People understand, and I let it go at that. Following this system I can even be brave enough at times to order shellfish or to poke around and ask for bread to sop up gravy. In general, bread is still something of a problem. It's still too much of a nuisance to try to butter it with a knife in the normal way. If the butter is in a little paper packet, I open it and rub the butter, it helps a lot if it's soft, across the bread. If the butter isn't soft, I take what I can get on the bread.

So don't be shy about using your fingers. Remember that asking is the key. I will often ask a friend I'm eating with if I have finished everything, if there is more meat left on the plate, and things like that. Choose desserts that are easy to eat. I don't order Napoleons, they're too flaky. It's easier to eat ice cream, many fruit desserts, or cake. You need to figure out what you want to handle by fork or by finger.

As I've been stressing throughout this book, having low vision is like being enrolled in a crash course in overcoming shyness. When my friends read the menu to me I ask prices, especially when I am paying for it. On the other hand you don't want to overburden those around you. So, for example, when it's a question of the menu, I try to avoid asking my friends to read the whole thing. Instead I'll say, "I feel like fish. What are the fish appetizers and entrees?" Or, very helpful: "I'll wait to see what the rest of you order." Then I wait and let them sift through the menu. They usually choose a reasonable selection, and it makes the whole affair quite easy and efficient for me.

I used to dump food and water on myself, on tablecloths, and on the floor until **I learned a few important rules:**

1. Find out where your wine or water glass is. When you pick it up, return it exactly to that spot.

2. Lean over your plate when you eat. Your posture will have to be a little less upright than you're probably used to, but your food and fork are over the dish.

3. Be generous with napkins. Get extras and put a couple of them under your chin and a couple more on your lap. If you have a cloth napkin, spread it across your chest in self-defense. This may not look elegant but it will save you a lot of cleaning bills and even more embarrassment.

4. If you've got a small plate of food, a salad maybe,
   put the plate on a larger plate so that what you spill
   falls on the big plate and not on the table or on you.
   (At home, you could use a tray.)

Despite all these precautions, sometimes you are just going to make a mess. I'm exuberant, I eat with my hands, but I also talk with my hands. One day I forgot where everything was and in my effervescence I knocked over a glass of water. I was mortified! Simply mortified! But there was nothing to do except apologize. The waiter simply cleared everything away and put down a fresh tablecloth. I learned right then and there, if you say you're sorry it's okay. You don't have to make excuses. As long as you're decent and pleasant about it, people understand.

Food on trains and airplanes is particularly hard to handle. Not only is there movement from time to time that you can't control, but often you can't choose things that are easy for you to eat. When I can choose in these situations, I tend to order "easy-eat" food. Sandwiches are easy-eat; so is soup. Though I love eggs over easy, I don't order them unless I'm in very comfortable surroundings. For the same reason, I avoid gloppy food like eggplant parmesan or quiche. Even if I can cut it with a knife and fork, or just a fork, it's hard to handle. In these situations I also try to use a fork only. A knife is an extension of your hand, like a paint brush, and if you can't see what you're doing, it is often hard to use.

Picnicking and other small pleasures simply depend on your mood and the willingness of people around you to help because they recognize your limitations and value your good friendship. At a picnic I'll ask for something easy to handle, like a hamburger. I'll skip the sparerib because I'd have to deal with the bone, which is difficult. These are the choices you make.

As always, however, each person is different and may find different solutions to these problems. One last tip to help you avoid trying to sip your soup with the bowl of the spoon upside down: usually the design of raised engraving is found only on the up side. If you examine the handle of the utensil before you dive in, you can determine the up side and avoid unnecessary spills.

What's useful for you here? What do you want to remember? What do you know that is as good or better as these suggestions?

Chapter 9
TRAVELING

Traveling to the corner, across town, or around the world are all experiences within the reach of many low vision people. But opportunities for travel are obviously going to be much more restricted than for sighted people.

Failing sight notwithstanding, after I retired I had the good fortune to be able to take trips, extended trips, out of the country once or twice a year so that over a nine-year period, little by little, I traveled around the world. Toward the end I was using my cane. Now, when I no longer do that kind of traveling because it's more difficult for me, I have wonderful memories that I can enjoy.

When you're traveling in a car or train you won't really be able to take in much of what's around you, and no one's going to give you a running commentary on everything out the window. So, you have to make it up. You have to take what you get, whatever that may be, and create a world within you that you relate, as best you can, to the world outside you.

The advantages of blindness: *it stimulates your creative imagination and excites your curiosity.*

PACKING

For efficiency and convenience, be a careful packer. Begin by packing as lightly as you can. I traveled around the world for months with one suitcase weighing only seventeen pounds. It can be done. The key is to think it through carefully. Run through the trip in your mind and decide what you will need, scene by scene, imagining all the possible activities and weather you're likely to encounter. Plan to wear layers to economize on weight and space and to pack versatile things that you can use over and over again for many different occasions. For example, I often take two skirts, two sweaters, and four blouses. These can be mixed and matched to make literally dozens of different outfits. Once, in Hong Kong, I used a dress as a blouse, just wearing a skirt over it. It's important to color-coordinate things so that you always look good. To this end, when I travel, I simplify the colors I take with me. I leave out most patterns as well as the reds, pinks, and oranges, which can easily clash. Instead, I keep to the tans and blues. It's less interesting but a lot safer and easier.

Here's a tip that will keep you from going crazy. When you pack put similar items together in individual plastic bags. For instance, put your underwear in one, night clothes in another, pharmaceuticals in a third. You may want to have individual plastic bags for each blouse or sweater, but put a matching outfit in a single bag. The advantage to this system is that you can put your hand on a given item quickly without having to go through the whole suitcase. This will vastly increase the amount of time you can spend doing fun things.

More tips to help you color-coordinate: pack items that you can recognize by texture. The nubby sweater is tan, the smooth one blue, the silk blouse white, the cotton blouse blue, and so on. Also, keep your pairs of shoes together in separate bags and roll into the shoes the socks or stockings that go with them. Not only does this last trick save space, it makes it easy for you to find the matching items when you want them.

TICKETS AND ACCOMMODATIONS

You've got to buy tickets for your trip and also book hotels. As a rule travel agents don't know the needs of low vision people. That's why I usually make my own arrangements.

First, I call the airline or railroad or bus company and speak directly to the ticketing people. I tell the agent my name, where and when I want to go, and that I have a disability. Then I explain my special needs, in detail. This assures me of easy accessibility to service on the train, plane, or bus.

GETTING TO THE TICKET COUNTER

Getting the tickets requires going to the ticket counter. A friendly person has to take you, although not necessarily a friend. You can get a skycap to do it at the airport, and you can get a cab driver to get you a skycap if you come by taxi. Whoever drives you needs to put you in the hands of someone else who can take you to the ticket counter. If you come by bus, it can be the bus driver, though sometimes another passenger will volunteer to do it. As always, be prepared to tip. It helps to have a tip ready in hand when you ask the skycap or porter to take you and your bag to the ticket counter.

IN THE TERMINAL AND ON THE PLANE OR TRAIN

Because I have called ahead, the airline (let's just stick with that as an example, but similar things could be said for other kinds of transportation) knows I am arriving and that I need help going from the ticket counter to the waiting area. They also know that I'll need an escort from the waiting room onto the plane and an attendant to take me to my seat. I have also explained that I will need the attendant to show me the location of the restroom as well as some other things, like where the toilet flush is and how to use the basin. She or he will have to show me how my meal is laid out on my tray and on the plates and perhaps even cut and help me with the food. The airline also knows that I need assistance getting off the plane, retrieving my luggage, and then getting to my local transportation.

All these services and attentions can be arranged if you call ahead and explain each phase in detail. It took me many years to lose the shame I felt at asking for such personal service. Now I get remarkable service, and you will too if you are pleasant and keep your requests to a minimum. I've found attendants on planes and trains most accommodating once I explained my disability. If the attendant escorts me to the bathroom, I'll have to ask them to wait for me or to keep an eye open for when I'm finished and ready to get back to my seat. If I have to stand in the aisle, the cane shows people that I am blind, which is a help to everyone. They can tell the attendant I'm waiting, or simply offer to help. A white cane and a Braille book are both, by the way, great conversation pieces, especially the book.

Sometimes when you are being escorted people will treat you, the blind person, as if you aren't there. I was being taken to the ramp at the airport by my daughter, and the flight attendant, utterly ignoring me, asked her, "Shall I take her bag onto the plane?" I interrupted and said, "Please. Talk to me. I'm blind, but I can still hear and talk, and I'm the one, after all, who's going on the plane. Thank you." Although I am always irritated by such treatment, I make it my business to add, "I know, of course, you were addressing my companion instead of me out of kindness." People do this quite unconsciously, I think. Unless people make eye contact with you, they tend not to address you, perhaps because they think you're not paying attention. Since I have been blind I've tried to remember to look at people as much as I can rather than stare into space like Homer. It helps. I guess I wasn't doing it that day at the airport, though. Of course, the flight attendant had just started to talk. From then on I had a relationship with her.

AT THE HOTEL

As with the airline, it's the same with the hotel. It's essential that you call ahead and alert the management to your special needs. This means that you've already arranged to be greeted at the curb. However, the message may not have made it to there, so once again when you arrive you may have to get help from your driver. Make sure that one caring service person passes you on to the next, just as you did in the airport. The cab driver puts you in the hands of the bellhop, for example. There's nothing so scary as being left alone in a strange place without being able to see what's around you. Even now, when a bellhop tells me "I'll be right back, ma'am," I have to struggle a little with my fear that I'll be forgotten. Of course that's part of the price of blindness, and I meet it as cheerfully as I can. I also try to prepare myself and those around me. So I get the bellhop, or whoever, to take me to the front desk, having made sure to ask him if the baggage is with him. If it is coming separately I ask who has it.

The same procedure applies for getting to your room. But not only must someone take you there, once you are in the room you must ask where everything is: lights, bureau, closet and hangers, window, heat and air conditioning switches, shower, tub, sink, toilet, sofa, luggage rack, and so on. You need to find out how the shower and the faucets work. But most of all, what you must know is where the phone is and how you get to the front desk.

TRAVELING ALONE VERSUS TRAVELING WITH A SIGHTED FRIEND

The difference between traveling alone and traveling with a sighted friend is that alone you have total independence, whereas traveling with a friend necessarily puts you in something of a dependent position. On the one hand this dependence is good, because you do need help. On the other hand, you lose some of your sense of being a psychologically autonomous grown-up. All of us want to have control over life's little details, where, when, and how things are done, and generally do for ourselves.

Here's an example of how you can lose your autonomy, and the feeling of dignity it provides, when traveling with a friend. This really happened to me. I called up the airline, arranged for the tickets and booked the seats I wanted, near the lavatory. But when I got to the plane, I discovered that my companion had also talked to the airline and had changed our seats. There was nothing I could do about it. It was a done thing. I felt frustration and anger. Sometimes I feel this way even if my companion has engineered a practical improvement, because I was not consulted. I was treated as a dependent. This sort of thing happens all the time when you're blind.

Another common example is when the porter at the airport insists you get into a wheelchair when you are able and want to walk. It's easier for him, so he dumps you in, further emphasizing your helplessness. Another example: While walking down the street my friend guides me toward the ramp at the curb crossing, thinking it's easier for me and saying, "We're about to go down the ramp." But it's actually easier for me to use the curb. If I use the ramp, I generally can't tell exactly when I'm in the roadway. But my companion doesn't know that. Normally I don't protest, but it's another little bit of wear and tear, isn't it? Or similarly, my companion might place my hand on a handrail, but I want to find it for myself.

I think it's normal for blind people to want to do all they can for themselves, by themselves. But helpful sighted people aren't perfect, or perfectly trained to deal with blindness. It would be much better, in fact, if they were trained to read our minds! Because this isn't the case, I urge myself and urge you to make compromises and adjustments. Seek the best balance between comfort and safety on the one hand, and complete independence on the other. So here is a rule of thumb: *The best guide is yourself. The best way to figure out what you need is to figure it out for yourself.* Then, when you have done that, you will be able to get the most out of having a sighted guide.

It would be ungenerous and wrong of me to end this section about traveling with a sighted friend on this note only. Obviously such travel has many advantages. One very important advantage is that the sighted person can make you acquainted with a new area in detail, orienting you for future visits. If, for instance, you stay at a hotel in some foreign city for a few days, your friend can walk out with you a couple of times and lay out the succession of shops on a particular street. Then you can visit them on your own later. For that matter, a friend can do the same in your own city, even in parts of your neighborhood that you don't know by heart.

TRAVELING WITH A BLIND FRIEND

On the other hand, traveling with a blind companion can be a rich and fulfilling experience. There is a possibility of a deep companionship. Only another blind person can fully understand the way we live and the world, the interior world, we live in. This makes traveling with a blind companion a worthwhile alternative, at appropriate times, to traveling alone or with someone sighted. The sighted person tends to think for you; on your own you're independent, but you're lonely. With a blind person you have someone with whom to talk out all your little dilemmas and problems, needs and idiosyncrasies. Traveling with a blind person, even for a walk of a few blocks, can be a great adventure. Daily life for the blind is always a series of little struggles and small victories. But the victory gets bigger, somehow, when shared solutions are created.

Just the other day I went out with a blind friend for the day in San Francisco. We did many of the things one does out of the home. We went to stores, to a bank, to a restaurant, and for a stroll. We might have been tourists, even though San Francisco is our own hometown. First, we made a date. Then we met and called a cab, rode to the first store we wanted to go to, made our way into the store with the help of someone outside, told the sales clerk we were blind, bought what we needed, asked for the location of a nearby restaurant, poked our way out of the store, found the restaurant, were served and ate lunch, paid our bill, and so forth. You can imagine the special sense of comfort and intimacy that many times arose between us during all of this. It's really quite different from being with a sighted companion. When the time came to pay the bill we were not dependent on anyone else. We each acted as independent individuals. Also, when we asked the waitress to read the bill to us, we each knew that two of us were listening. We were part of an "us," and that goes such a long way not just toward relieving loneliness but also toward relieving those feelings of deep isolation, strangeness, even shame that come from being different from everyone else. When we paid the bill, each of us took out our money (organized according to our individual systems for folding bills), paid our half and then left our half of the tip. Inevitably, we shared a sense of achievement.

It was the same when we came to take our walk later in the afternoon. We moved slowly, block after block, downtown, deciding how to get to the corner, whether to go to the left or the right, working out each obstacle, each crossing, listening for the clanging of the cable car, hearing it go by, listening for the traffic to stop, my taking his arm or hand, moving my cane out in front of us to be visible to drivers. At one intersection we waited twice for the traffic to stop because the first time we weren't ready. It is necessary to be poised to move the moment the light changes in our favor, because we need the whole time between lights to make our way across the street. I wouldn't be doing things this way were I traveling with a sighted person who's protecting me. But that's the way we do it.

So that's who we were, two blind people working it out, getting around by working together. "Jim," I said at one point, "I feel something soft under my foot. I believe it's something like a drop cloth. What do you make of it?" "Yes. I think you're right, there's an obstacle, let's move to the left until we're past it," and we did. Then we advanced again. I, poking and tapping with the cane, located the scaffolding and found our way around it. To the sighted person observing us we didn't look outrageous. Instead, we looked like two people who are simply slow and don't see very well, dignified and purposeful, but not odd or bizarre. This self-image gives us an added sense of satisfaction in our competence.

We went past the scaffolding and came to a traffic tunnel. Jim recognized where we were, found the stairway for pedestrians that climbs over it, and we went up. I wiped the handrail in my usual way and measured the height of the steps. At the top we knew which way to turn because Jim knew this territory. We were headed toward the corner of Mason and Taylor and a particular barber shop. Here, I asked for help. "Can you see the barber shop from here?" I asked a passerby, who stopped and replied: "Yeah. It's down the way you're going toward the middle of the block. About eight stores." The last piece of information didn't mean much to us, but now we knew it was about in the middle of the block, so when we got about that far, Jim said, "I think we're here." And I replied, "I think so, too." So we poked around and found an opening of a store and then we listened. "This sounds like the barber shop," he said, and in we went.

Later on we wanted to go to a record store. Well, your other senses don't expand with vision loss, but you do learn to use them in a different way. Jim said, as we poked our heads into one place, "No, this doesn't smell like a record store." And he was right. We all know that the sounds and smells of a record store are different from those of a clothing store, and that a supermarket smells and sounds different than a delicatessen. But only blind people need to use this knowledge purposefully.

That's the way of it: that's how two blind people make their way around a city, asking for help along the way but not leaning on anyone in particular. The only real personal assistance I needed was getting into the barber's chair without breaking my neck falling over the foot rest. If I had been walking with a sighted person it all would have gone more quickly. But, in a way, I would have been dumb as well as blind. The other person would have determined the course, the changes in direction, distances, and all the rest, leaving me out of any active thinking. Kind of like the man I mentioned before who was pulled across the street in Washington D.C. by the tip of his cane like a donkey. He had to submit and in doing so he had to give up a lot of his sense of self.

Chapter 10
MEMORY

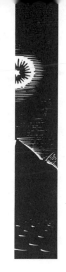

When I'm home I tend to put my glasses down and forget where they are. It's really a game I play with myself because I don't think about where I'm putting them, but there are four places in which these glasses can be found and most likely I'll find them in one of these places. Why I don't remember where I put my glasses, I don't know. Maybe I don't remember because the glasses don't do me very much good, but nevertheless they are a crutch, and nevertheless I am deliberately forgetful. However, I am not so deliberately forgetful of where I put my house keys, because that would be a very serious matter if I put them down carelessly and then had to look all over the place and maybe not even find them. The fact is if you look in the last place first you'll save yourself a lot of wear and tear. In our case, if you can't see, out of sight is indeed out of mind. Eyesight is truly the first large element of memory, of remembering. But since we don't have it or not much of it we need to turn around and solve our problems in a different way.

My solution is to equate memory with learning. You learn something and so you remember it. *You remember it for as long as you need it. Then you drop it entirely, or you put it on the back burner, or you put it in your bank vault.* Those are the three kinds of memory. Improving your memory is actually what this chapter is all about. I'm not considering memory loss or forgetfulness as an aspect of a physical ailment such as a diagnosed illness. I'm talking about remembrance and learning retention for people whose sight is failing and need to use four senses instead of five to get on with the business of living.

When a low vision person is introduced to somebody, we can't see them. We hear the name and we'll say, "I didn't quite catch your name. What is your name? How do you spell your name?" There's no shame in saying this. As a matter of fact, we're ahead of the game because sighted people are ashamed to use such a device in order to try to get a stranger's name. We can do it. We can be graceful about it and it's accepted. As a matter of fact my sighted friends will say, "I don't know so and so's name." I'll say, "Oh, never you mind, I'll find out for you." When the person comes over I, the one who cannot see, finds it easy and appropriate and acceptable to say, "Who are you? Tell me your name again." Then my sighted friend, at that point, is on the alert and knows the name. So you see, that's one of the advantages of not seeing. We can help out. We can easily ask for repetition of name, address, phone number, or whatever it is we need without feeling ashamed and without feeling the person that we're asking feels that we're being stupid. He simply accepts the fact that as an unsighted person we need repetition of information, and it's acceptable for the reason that since we don't see facial expressions and body language, we need to strengthen our memory in our own peculiar ways. In our own special ways of learning I should say.

MEMORY AIDS AND TECHNIQUES

Diminished sight will lead to forgetfulness unless you recognize the problem and work on it. First of all, as I mentioned earlier in this book, get a hand-held tape recorder and learn to use it. I like to keep a small hand-held tape recorder at my telephone. I can talk into the machine as I'm talking to the person on the telephone. I use it to remind myself of appointments, for phone numbers or whatever it is that I need to remember. I even put my grocery list on it so that when I am ready to go out, I can write on a piece of paper what my list is and hand it to the person at the store to help me. You see the things I'm suggesting you put on that tape recorder are things that you want to remember for a little while. Then you drop it, erase the tape and start all over.

Anything that you want to remember for a longer time *(the back burner)* you probably need to store in a different way, possibly on a second tape recorder. You may want a list of all the theater events or movies that you want to see in the next month or two. So that's on a different tape for longer term remembering. Maybe that's the tape on which you put your flight number for a trip you're taking two months from now, for instance.

Then maybe you'll want a special recorder, a third one, for long term memory *(the bank vault)*. Things like telephone numbers are a long term memory example. It's possible to use three different tapes with the same recorder. For myself I've learned from experience that I'm better off buying three cheap tape recorders than juggling cassettes. I usually put a bit of Scotch tape on side one of any cassette I use. If you're going to juggle cassettes, you might try putting one piece of Scotch tape on your first, two bits of Scotch tape on the second, and three bits of tape on the third. You can make up your own system for this. You might use rubber bands, or maybe a series of those little adhesive dots that you can buy in the hardware store.

I never leave home without a hand-held tape recorder and, as a matter of fact, a talking clock slipped into my pocket or purse. Sighted people are always amazed and amused by the gadgets that low vision persons carry with them. They're curious and quite surprised at how well we get along.

For the house there are many kinds of talking or musical clocks that will keep you company and well-advised of the time. If you're lucky enough to have a Westminster clock, you'll hear it chime every fifteen minutes. Musical clocks will strike the half hour. Then there are clocks you can simply touch for the time at that very moment. Some clocks have daily calendars on them as well. Then there are clocks and calendars that are part of a small calculator setup. So if you're willing to learn these things, you're at no loss at all.

Kitchen timers are wonderful reminders for sighted as well as non sighted people. You can set them to remind you to turn off the oven, or switch on your favorite radio program. You can use it when you want to nap. Another aid in these days of new electronic gadgets is the answering machine on your phone. You can learn to use your answering machine and leave messages for yourself on it.

You can be in better shape than sighted people if you learn to keep your environment organized and keep your materials in expected, logical places. Keys belong in pockets or around the door knob as you walk out of the house. Shoes belong two by two, like twins, either on the floor of your closet or in shoe bags or whatever. They can be organized not only in twosies, being pairs, but also arranged by color. Sometimes you can't identify the color of the shoe by shape or feel because you may have several shoes of the same type. But if they're so arranged that black shoes are with black shoes and brown, etc., you won't go wrong. And even with shoes you don't have to remember about left and right. With lace shoes put a knot in your right hand lace.

People often say to me, "Oh, you're so well put together. The colors you're wearing are so nice. How do you do it?" I do it by putting garments that go together on the same hanger. Learn the textures of your clothing so you can tell a nubby cotton from a wool from a polyester, and so on. If you keep the "go-togethers" together you won't have any trouble. In your dresser drawers you simply remember where your undergarments are, where your socks are, and so on. It doesn't have anything to do with seeing. If they're always in the same place there will be no trouble at all.

This is the sort of learning that, once done, you no longer have to think about. There are other kinds of memory that you might be worrying about. Maybe you're afraid of being forgetful in general. You don't have to be forgetful if you just develop some good techniques for remembering. One of the best techniques is your tape recorder. If you forget a phone number or a recipe, you have it on cassette tape. I'll put a recipe on tape as a friend of mine tells it to me. The best way to do this, I've discovered, is to use short ten minute tapes and record a single recipe on one side of the tape. This way I don't have to go back and forth looking for a particular recipe. It's on a ten minute tape, and I have it in a little holder. This is my talking cookbook.

There are all kinds of learning gimmicks like the proverbial string around the finger that you can use to help you remember things. I keep a little plant in a very special place to remind me to water all the other plants. If you want to remember Mr. Jones, you might say Mr. Jones and Mr. Bones to help. Or I'll remember the name of my next door neighbor because his name is like my name. His name is Frank and my name is Frances. Sometimes I make a jingle out of what I want to buy in the store. For instance, "Milk and meat and jam would be neat." Any kind of silliness that appeals to you is good enough. Once I made up a whole set of silly words and when I got to the store I knew the silly words but forgot what the silly words were meant to be. You might string words together in some sentence that sounds like nonsense but will remind you of what you want to do. Or you might make up a word out of the initial letters of a number of words, an acronym.

However, there are circumstances in which your tape recorder will not help you, where you must rely on your own resources to remember. One way to get around successfully and know where you are is to develop active observation. We need to actively observe as we explore new terrain, new situations, new environments, and so on. For example, I can find my way to the doctor's office because I have observed its "landmarks" carefully. There are steps going up from the outside hall and then steps going down into the office, and the office is dark. Over to the left there is a chair, and over to the right there is a couch. I actually, unknowingly, sat in a gentleman's lap on the couch once, but gracefully apologized by explaining my situation. In meeting and greeting people, whether you know them or not, the only hint you have as to who they are is the voice. Again you approach it gracefully. "I know the voice but I can't place it, who are you?" So you see, to remember things we need to be very active, conscious, and observant. It's much more work than if you could see, but this is our lot in life and we face it and act on it the best we can.

Do you ever walk along the street mumbling to yourself about this and that? One day I was walking along talking to myself when a gentleman came up to me and said, "Madam, if you're talking to yourself that's one thing, but if you're talking to me, would you please speak up?" Well, you can either be embarrassed about something like this or you can laugh and say, "You've got a point there." Or you can explain, "This is my way of remembering things." We all devise different ways to remember.

I'll remember a phone number by the design it makes on my touch-tone phone. Maybe you can do that. A number like 3-6-9-6, for example, is easy because I know that three, six, and nine follow each other down the right-hand side. I do this quite often and quite successfully. My own personal telephone directory is a Voxcom, a series of index cards with a magnetic strip on them which I can run through a small machine that talks out to me, one card at a time, the name, address, and phone number of each person in my phone book. I also have in it my social security number, my credit card number, and so on. This device can be found in any one of a number of catalogs of materials for the blind, or in stores that deal with items for low vision people.

If you're going marketing I previously suggested a hand-held tape recorder from which you transpose your list onto a piece of paper, then hand it to a customer service person in the store.

The same technique will work for a doctor's appointment. If you have questions, you do what you did when you were sighted, you jot down the things you want to know. You can't very well jot them down on paper, but you can bring your tape recorder and say, "These are the things I need to know." There's no shame in this. People need to address people with their needs. What you think of as loss of memory may very well have to do with tension and emotional discomfort. Don't jump to the conclusion that you're developing Alzheimer's disease just because you're forgetful. Of course Alzheimer's is a very serious disease, whose onset symptom is loss of memory. But consider that because your sight is diminishing, you're becoming more tense. Learning and remembering are related to a state of well-being, relaxation, and emotional health.

Medication is another factor that may sometimes affect memory. Alcohol consumption is another factor to look at. One glass of wine a day won't harm most people, but a lot more will, very often, affect your memory.

Keep your life simple, keep your wits about you, and know that there are certain things that must be learned. For instance, I have a new toaster oven. It took me several hours with a patient person to teach me how to use the oven. Now I know how to use it. It has nothing to do with memory, it has to do with learning. The same thing with the television. I can't see the channel numbers on it, but I have the television dial marked so that I can get from one channel to another without having to listen in order to figure out which it is. It's the same thing with the washer, the dryer, and the stove. They are marked so that I know how to use them. It's at your discretion that the items in your house are marked for your use, for your logic.

Being nervous when you're learning something will militate against you. Take it easy. It's natural to tense up if you're on a bus or a train or in a restaurant, but you really will learn to handle these situations. There are times when you rely on the kindness of the people around you. For example, when eating, remember that a fork is usually to the left and a knife is usually to the right and that a water glass is a hazard and ask where it is. Then if people are going to be putting things on your plate, request to put one item on at a time so you don't become confused. And I say it clearly with no shame because that is the name of the game. That is, it's the name of the game for me. The idea is to avoid disorientation and confusion by keeping things simple, remembering some things, learning others, and asking for help when you know that you need it.

So if you worry about the word "memory," I'd forget it and pick up the words *remembering* or *learning,* because I believe sincerely that that's what is truly meant. Memory retention can clutter your head with all sorts of things that you really don't need, but if you learn situations, you learn environments, you'll do very well. Keeping yourself active to the limit of your strength, and keeping to a schedule that is comfortable for you, is a matter of developing good mental health practices. Good mental health practices will do very well for you in remembering things, in appetite, in sleeping, in making the best of your life. There may be things that you can no longer do like participating in sports, but you can probably find alternatives that provide the same satisfaction and effect. These days I can't cut glass for my stained glass hobby. But if I could get somebody to square up a piece of paper for me, I could make the design. Some people crochet and knit, even though they can't see. Some low vision and blind people even paint. They use the textures in their materials to help them identify color, shape, and so on. No one ever promised us a rose garden. Each one of us has to cultivate our own.

Sighted people are at an advantage. It takes low vision people a longer time to differentiate the three basic types of memory: *1) instant recall memory; 2) back burner memory; 3) bank vault memory,* and apply our learned memory aids to assist, but we can. We need to take in things with four senses instead of five.

One blind young woman I know came into a house, went over to the wall and reached up high to feel the wall and reached down low to feel the floor, so that she would understand the baseboards, the type of walls and so on. Touch things to learn them. Of course, ask first if you may. Memory is a learning process of holding, filing, and assimilating the information you need for your journey of life.

Out of chaos, comes organized confusion. Out of organized confusion comes rationality. This rationality leads down other paths to successful and satisfying new ways of life. Enjoy your journey of *dancing in the dark.*

AFTERWORD

When I first saw my mother at a large family affair, after not seeing her for quite a few years, I was surprised and amazed by her. She had virtually no sight left, yet to me, appeared to make contact with others and handle herself in a way I'd never seen before.

Her loss of vision was masked by (I would never have taken her for a blind person, had I not known) her ability to follow you with her eyes and at the same time be witty and charming in a most relaxed manner. This woman did not seem uncomfortable with herself nor draw any special attention as you might think she would. "Can she actually not see?" I asked myself.

I'd never seen her so gracious and at ease! The delicate grace she exhibited when reaching for the food from the buffet stunned me. Never had I seen such determination and deliberation in her eating pattern.

Mom had grown up! She had become her own person. Although some may feel sorry for her and wish this thing had never happened to her, I have to admit that never have I felt so proud or close to her. So, for me, this blind thing has been a good thing. And I know it has been for my mother too. All the experiences she has had, and the knowledge and things she had to learn about herself and others, would probably never had occurred had she not lost her vision.

Amy Hunter
Mt. Kisco, NY
October, 1993

THE DICK AND JANE PRIMER OF COMMON EYE DISORDERS

Sponsored by: The Department of Ophthalmology, University of California Medical Center, San Francisco, Dr. Steven G. Kramer, Dr. William V. Good, (medical advisors)

The American Academy of Ophthalmology says low vision "is when ordinary eye glasses or contact lenses are unable to bring a person's sight up to normal."

Definitions

This section contains simple descriptions of a few conditions that can cause loss of vision or blindness. Here are some medical words that need some explanation.

Ophthalmologist

A doctor who treats the eye and is an eye surgeon.

Optometrist

A person trained to examine eyes and prescribe glasses. Although optometrists often test for eye disease, they are not trained to treat them.

Optician

A person who makes glasses.

Optical Aids

Things you can use to help you see better, like eyeglasses, magnifying lenses and other kinds of enlargers.

Laser

A powerful beam of light which can sometimes be used to cut or seal tissue without surgery.

Peripheral Vision

Vision to the left, right, above and below what you are looking at.

Cornea

The thin clear tissue which is the front of the eyeball.

Vitreous

The clear gel inside the eyeball. It keeps the eyeball's shape and allows light to pass through.

Pupil

The black spot in the center of the eyeball. It is actually a hole, covered by the cornea, through which light passes.

Iris

The colored circle around the pupil that changes the size of the pupil for different light conditions.

The lens is just behind the pupil. It focuses what you see on the retina at the back of the eye.

Retina

A nerve tissue in the back of the eye. It catches the light that has passed through the lens and sends it on to the brain where it becomes pictures.

Macula

The macula is in the center of the retina. It gives us forward vision, allowing us to read and to see exactly what things look like.

Optic Nerve

The optic nerve connects the retina to the brain. It is the path that the light captured by the retina travels on its way to the brain.

Common Eye Disorders

Cataracts

Condition

A cataract is like a clouding of the lens of the eye. When the lens is clear, it passes light to the retina. Sometimes the clouding continues for a long time before you know your sight is changing. A cataract can cause hazy or foggy vision. The pupil, which is normally black, can turn yellowish or cloudy white.

Cause

There are many kinds of cataracts. The most common is the kind that develop as we grow older, starting at about age 40. This is called a senile cataract.

Sometimes babies are born with cataracts. This kind of cataract is called a congenital cataract. When these cataracts are treated immediately, the baby's sight is saved. Neglect leads to blindness.

Another kind of cataract happens from an accident to the eye, like hitting it, poking it, or cutting it. This is called a traumatic cataract.

Sometimes other diseases, like diabetes, can start a cataract. This is called a secondary cataract.

Care

So far, the only thing that can cure a cataract is surgery. Ask your ophthalmologist about medicine, eye drops, or other treatments that you think might be good for you.

Cure

Almost all cataract operations are successful; but there is always risk with any surgery. In cataract surgery, the cloudy lens is taken out.

Once the lens is removed, your eye needs a substitute lens. This could be special cataract glasses, contact lenses, or permanent artificial lenses put in the eye.

Sometimes it takes a long time for good sight to return. Talk to your ophthalmologist about the best method for you.

For safety's sake, it can never hurt to keep your head above your heart after eye surgery. Avoid bending over after eye surgery until your ophthalmologist says your eye has completely healed.

Macular Degeneration

Condition
Macular degeneration is a breakdown of sight in the retina. The macula is part of the retina. You might notice a dark or empty spot when you look at something. Sometimes, if macular degeneration happens only in one eye, you don't even know there's a dark or empty spot, because the other eye is doing the work of two eyes.

Cause
Most of the time, macular degeneration is caused by a thinning or breakdown of the retina around the macula. Sometimes, the blood vessels break down and scar tissue blocks your sight.

Care and Coping
As the macula becomes weaker, or degenerates, you will find reading and close-up work harder for you. The way you see colors may change. When you feel your sight is changing, the best thing to do is visit your ophthalmologist right away.

You may find different ways to make it easier to see, such as magnifying glasses and brighter lights. Your library has machines that magnify anything you want to read. They have large-print books and even "talking books." Ask the librarian about other things they may have for low-vision people.

Cure
There is no cure for macular degeneration. In a few cases, early in the disorder, laser surgery may help. It is important to visit you ophthal-

mologist right away when you notice a change in your sight.

Glaucoma

Condition

At first, glaucoma affects your vision above, below, and to the sides of what you are looking at. This is called peripheral vision. Glaucoma may give you tunnel vision, where you can see straight ahead, but not to the left or right, or up or down.

Fluid pressure builds up in the eye and causes pressure against the nerves. This happens because the fluid inside the eyeball can't drain out of the eye. The drain in the eye is called a canal. Imagine a wash-cloth blocking the drain of your bathtub, and the water staying in the tub and not being able to drain out. That is what it is like when the canal of your eye is blocked and the fluid cannot drain out. The pressure from the fluid damages the optic nerve. The nerve is important because it connects the eye to the brain. Glaucoma is usually slow and painless and is known as "the silent enemy."

Cause

Most of the time glaucoma happens because the drainage canals are blocked. Usually the block is mild. The fluid drains out more slowly and your eyesight changes very slowly. Sometimes the canal is blocked very suddenly and the pressure builds up very quickly. Then you might feel pain or become nauseated and your sight will be blurred. You might even become blind in a day. Put in an emergency call to your eye clinic or ophthalmologist right away.

Care

Glaucoma can generally be treated if found in the early stages. It does not usually lead to blindness. Eye drops and/or pills are usually used to treat glaucoma. If you have side effects from the medicine, tell your ophthalmologist. Sometimes laser treatment can be used to reduce the pressure in the eye. Sometimes surgery can also be used to make new drainage openings.

For safety's sake, it can never hurt to keep your head above your heart after eye surgery. Avoid bending over until your ophthalmologist says your eye has completely healed.

Cure

There is no cure for glaucoma. Treatment can keep the disorder under control and prevent most loss of sight, however, the best cure is prevention; the best prevention is eye exams. The common rule is: an eye exam every year after age 40.

Diabetic Retinopathy

Condition

Diabetic retinopathy is a combination of two words. It means that a person with diabetes may have a disorder in the retina. Diabetes affects blood sugar levels.

Blood sugar levels affect the blood vessels in the retina. The blood vessels change size and sometimes leak.

Cause

The exact cause of diabetic retinopathy is not understood. Diabetes, however, seems to cause a weakening of the capillaries (very small blood vessels) all over the body. Pregnancy or high blood pressure often make this condition worse.

There are two types of diabetic retinopathy. In background retinopathy the blood vessels within the retina change. This is an early stage of diabetic retinopathy. Sight is usually not seriously affected and the disorder does not get worse in about 80% of diabetic people with the disorder.

A second, more advanced form of retinopathy is called proliferative retinopathy. This begins the same way as background retinopathy. The fragile new blood vessels break and bleed into the vitreous (the clear fluid in the eye). This blood causes the fluid to become cloudy, which blurs vision. Also, scar tissue forms, which tightens and pulls on the retina. This may pull the retina away from the tissue behind it (retinal detachment).

Blood vessels may also abnormally form in the iris, which can cause a type of glaucoma. Blindness may result from these conditions.

Care and Coping

Sometimes treatment for diabetic retinopathy is not necessary, especially with background retinopathy where vision is not affected. Only your ophthalmologist can tell. Other times, however, eye treatment is necessary to stop the disorder or improve vision. A very important treatment is "laser treatment." This means a surgeon directs a short burst of light which seals leaking blood vessels and forms small scars. These small scars reduce the abnormal vessel growth and help connect or attach the retina back to the eye. Laser treatment may help stop the damage, even in advanced cases. Remember, this method may not help you. It depends on the size and location of the damage, and how much the vitreous is clouded with blood.

In some cases, other surgery might help. A surgical procedure called a vitrectomy removes the vitreous and replaces it with an artificial clear solution. About 70% of vitrectomy patients have improved sight.

For safety's sake, it can never hurt to keep your head above your heart after eye surgery. Avoid bending over until your ophthalmologist says your eye has completely healed.

There is no cure for diabetes or diabetic retinopathy. Keeping diabetes under control and preventing loss of sight is generally possible. Successful treatment depends upon early diagnosis, taking all the medicines, and following the self-care recommended by your ophthalmologist.

Retinitis Pigmentosa

Condition

Retinitis pigmentosa is a hereditary disease that affects vision. It usually is first noticed by patients in childhood. The earliest symptoms are not being able to see in the dark and loss of peripheral vision (which is side vision).

Cause

Retinitis pigmentosa is caused by abnormal cells in the retina. Retinitis pigmentosa means a darker color in the cells in the retina. Males have this disorder more often than females. The disorder develops slowly over the years, and often does not lead to very low vision, since central vision (vision in the front) is the last to be affected. Sometimes people with this condition can see well for most of their lives; other times, people with this condition go blind.

Care and Coping

There is no treatment known to stop retinitis pigmentosa. Many aids are available to improve vision affected by retinitis pigmentosa. Some of these include special lenses to expand peripheral vision. Other mechanical and electronic devices may also work for you. Ask your ophthalmologist or clinic for information.

Cure

There is no cure for retinitis pigmentosa.

If there is any change in your eyesight run, don't walk, to your nearest ophthalmologist.

Appendix B
RESOURCE DIRECTORY

This directory is to be used as a resource and a motivating tool for you to do your own research on the agencies in your hometown. The author and publisher does not take responsibility for the information received from these agencies. It is highly recommended that you exercise common sense and careful thought before you follow any advice you may receive. The author gives full copyright permission to reprint and adapt this directory to suit your individual needs.

Section 1. Listening In

In Touch: Satellite Radio, Radio Broadcast for the Blind Program
15 West 65th Street, New York, NY. 10023
This radio station is on the air 24 hours a day, 7 days a week. In order to hear these radio programs you will need a special receiver.

Descriptive Video Service
To make TV more accessible to the visually impaired, contact your local public television station.

Telephone Company
Call your business office for FREE services for the blind.

Public Library/Communications Center
Contact your local library for talking books on cassette tapes and records are available FREE to borrow. You may also request a FREE cassette or record player. Ask for a bibliography of book and magazine titles on tape or soft disc recording.

California State Library   **(800) 952-5666**
Braille and talking book library.

Recordings for the Blind   **(415) 493-3717**
Scholarly library. Textbooks are available. Books can be recorded for you on special order.

Choice Magazine Listening
85 Channel Drive, Port Washington, NY. 11050
Selections from national magazines on cassette tapes FREE of charge.

Matilda Ziegler Magazine
20 West 17th Street, New York, NY. 10011   **(212) 242-0263**
Selections from national magazines on cassette tapes FREE of charge.

Section 2. Hands-On Exhibits

Botanical Gardens and Arboretums
These gardens of diverse fragrant plants is a delight for low vision and blind people.

Art Museums and Sculpture Gardens
Check out your local art museums and Sculpture Gardens for any special docent tours.

Zoo
Call ahead for appointment. The Zoos provide guides.

Historical Sites and Landmarks
Call for tour reservations or additional information.

Section 3. Organized Recreation

Environmental Traveling Companions (ETC)   **(415) 474-7662**
Year-round wilderness outings and environmental education experiences for people with special needs.

The Lighthouse   **(415) 431-1481**
Adult activities and classes. Enchanted Hills Summer Camp.

Murals in City Areas and Highways
Take a nice auto trip with a sighted friend.

V.I.P. Forum: Department of Ophthalmology,
University of California Medical Center
San Francisco, CA.   (415) 626-5313
Monthly medical discussions in the Bay Area

Section 4.   Going to the Dogs, Cats and Other Animals

Guide Dogs for the Blind, Inc.   (415) 499-4000
Provides guide dogs and the training in their use.

SPCA
Contact the one in your hometown for adoption of pets.

Section 5. Getting Around

American Foundation for the Blind   (415) 392-4845
This national advocacy organization offers an identification card to low vision people.

Paratransit Broker in your area
Taxi vouchers. Call for an application for all paratransit services, taxi, lift vans and group vans.

Department of Motor Vehicles
State identification card and disabled person parking placard issued.

Rapid Transit Company in Your Area for Bus or Train Services.

Section 6. Education

The Blind Babies Foundation, San Francisco, CA.   (415) 863-5464
Education, support groups and consultation for the parents of blind babies through preschool.

School for the Blind in Your State
Each state has at least one blind school, on primary and secondary levels.

State Department of Rehabilitation
Services offered include instruction in braille, typing, homemaking, daily living skills, and independent travel. The vocational rehabilitation program consists of job preparation services, including vocational counseling and evaluation, medical consultations, job training and placement.

109

State Department of Special Education
Check your State Department of Education.

Office of Services to the Blind, State Department of Social Services
Information and referral hotline; counseling by telephone. Blind awareness training upon request.

Your City's Public School District
Call for information concerning instruction on preschool elementary, and secondary levels.

Veterans Administration, Rehabilitation center
Check your local telephone directory. Residential facility for veterans.

San Francisco State University, Department of Special Education, Visually Handicapped Section
Contact: Dr. Sally Mangold, Chairperson   **(415) 338-1080**
The University offers low vision graduate programs as well as other disabling conditions. Through the Disabled Student Services Office assistance is available offering tutorial services as well as reading educational material onto tape for blind students.

Section 7. Educational Materials

American Foundation for the Blind
San Francisco, CA   **(415) 392-4845**
                                                 or (800) 232-5463
Directory of agencies serving the blind. Call for complete listings.

American Printing House for the Blind
PO Box 6085, Louisville, KY. 40206
Free catalog of educational materials, cassette players, and other visual aids.

Exceptional Teaching Aids
2010 Woobine Avenue, Castro Valley, CA. 94560   (510) 582-4859
Educational materials and equipment for visually impaired students.

National Association for Visually Handicapped,
San Francisco, CA.   **(415) 221-3201**
Large print books and low vision aids.

Section 8. Support Groups and Counseling

This organizations offer professional and peer counseling as well as crisis intervention.

The Lighthouse   Check your Yellow Pages.

Section 9. Low Vision Medical Services

These are groups offering information and assessments in this section. These specialized low vision services offer eye evaluation and how to use low vision aids.

American Academy of Ophthalmology
San Francisco, CA.   **(415) 775-5259**

National Eye Care Project
San Francisco, CA.   **(800) 222-3937**

Section 10.   Optical Aids and Computer Hardware

Innovative Rehabilitation Technology, Inc.,
Mountain View, CA.   **(415) 961-3161**
Audio and visual aids. Monthly magazine on cassette.

Your Local Utility Company
FREE highlighting or brailled knobs for your home appliances.

Science Products for the Blind
Box 385, Wayne, PA. 19087   **(800) 888-7400**
Manufactures and sells special scientific instruments. Gift and novelty items catalog available.

Sensory Access Foundation
Palo Alto, CA.   **(415) 329-0430**
This non-profit corporation adapts working environments and, using adaptive devices and sensory aids, prepares one for job placement. Catalog available.

Smith-Kettlewell Institute of Visual Sciences Rehabilitation
Engineering Services, San Francisco, CA.   **(415) 561-1620**
Recommends, prefabricates or adapts devices to meet specific needs.

Telesensory Systems, Inc.
Mountain View, CA.   **(415) 960-0920**
Manufactures and sells the Optacon, Speech-Plus and the Versa Braille.
Free catalog.

Section 11. Repair Services

Telephone Pioneers of America   Check your Yellow Pages.
Custom-made aids for persons with special needs. Repairs, replacements,
and adaptive aids.

Section 12. Home Care

The following agencies provide home care services for visually impaired
persons. Check your local phone book for home care services in your area.

Catholic Charities

Jewish Family and Children's Service

Meals on Wheels

Section 13. Legislation and Legal Action

American Civil Liberties Union (ACLU)   **(415) 621-2488**
Legal aid referral. In some cases will help you draft letters.

Legal Assistance to the Elderly, Inc.   **(415) 861-4444**
Lawyer referral for any matters relating to the elderly.

Section 14. Freebies

The following agencies and organizations offer FREE resource directories,
catalogs, newsletters, pamphlets and magazines. This is a partial List.

RESOURCE DIRECTORIES:

Federal Information Center   **(800) 726-4995**
Lists all federal agencies by subject, name, and phone number.

CATALOGS:

National Braille Press
88 St. Stephens Street, Boston, MA. 92115   (617) 266-6160

Lighthouse Low Vision Products
36-20 Northern Blvd., Long Island City, NY. 11101   (800) 453-4923

Mind's Eye, Box 1060
Petaluma, CA. 94953   (800) 227-2020

Pacifica Foundation
PO Box 8092, DEPT. A,
Universal City, CA. 91608-0092   (800) 735-0230

Royal National Institute for the Blind
Customer Service, PO Box 173
Peterborough PE 2-OWS England

Resources for Rehabilitation
33 Bedford Street, Suite 19A
Lexington, MA. 02173   (617) 862-6455
Telesensory
455 North Bernardo Ave
Mountain View, CA. 94039   (800) 227-8418

Victory Technology, INC.
425 Bush Street, San Francisco, CA. 94108   (800) 845-7737

Xerox/Kurzweil Personal Reader   (800) 762-4605

NEWSLETTERS:

California Council of Citizens with Low Vision   (800) 221-6359

GLEAMS, Foundation for Glaucoma Research   (415) 986-3162

LANTERN, The Lighthouse   (415) 431-1481

PAMPHLETS:

American Academy of Ophthalmology   (415) 561-8500
Pamphlets describing eye disorders

113

National Eye Institute
Bldg. 31, Room 6A32, Bethesda, MD. 20205
List of brochures on eye disorders available.

University of Maryland School of Pharmacy
20 North Pine street, Baltimore, MD. 21201
Booklets regarding your medicines available.

MAGAZINES:

Choice Magazine Listening
PO Box 10, Port Washington, NY. 11050   **(516) 883-8280**

Matilda Ziegler Magazine
20 West 17th Street, New York, NY. 10011   **(212) 242-0263**

Your local library/communication center for books on tape.

I am glad to be of assistance to you, I hope this information will help you find the agencies and services that will best serve you.

Frances Lief Neer

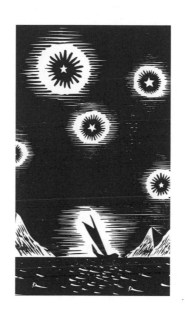